Instructor's Manual and Testbank to Accompany

CLINICAL DRUG THERAPY

RATIONALES FOR NURSING PRACTICE

i

Instructor's Manual and Testbank to Accompany

Clinical Drug Therapy

RATIONALES FOR NURSING PRACTICE

SIXTH EDITION

Anne Collins Abrams, RN, MSN
Associate Professor, Emeritus
Department of Baccalaureate and Graduate Nursing
College of Health Sciences
Eastern Kentucky University
Richmond, Kentucky

Gail Ropelewski-Ryan, RN, MSN
Nurse Education, Health, Physical Education and Recreation
Corning Community College
Corning, New York

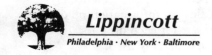

Lippincott
Philadelphia · New York · Baltimore

Ancillary Editor: Doris S. Wray
Project Editor: Erika Kors
Senior Production Manager: Helen Ewan
Senior Production Coordinator: Pat McCloskey
Art Director: Carolyn O'Brien
Manufacturing Manager: William Alberti

ISBN: 0-7817-2560-7

Any procedure or practice described in this book should be applied by the health care practitioner under appropriate supervision in accordance with professional standards of care used with regard to the unique circumstances that apply in each practice situation. Care has been taken to confirm the accuracy of information presented and to describe generally accepted practices. However, the authors, editors, and publisher cannot accept any responsibility for errors or omissions or for any consequences from application of the information in this book and make no warranty, express or implied, with respect to the contents of the book. Every effort has been made to ensure drug selections and dosages are in accordance with current recommendations and practice. Because of ongoing research, changes in government regulations, and the constant flow of information on drug therapy, reactions, and interactions, the reader is cautioned to check the package insert for each drug for indications, dosages, warnings, and precautions, particularly if the drug is new or infrequently used.

OVERVIEW

This manual has two main purposes. One purpose is to facilitate the use of *Clinical Drug Therapy: Rationales for Nursing Practice*. The second purpose is to assist the instructor in evaluating students' knowledge of drug information and their ability to apply that information in client-care situations.

To fulfill the first purpose, assorted teaching materials are presented so the instructor can choose those most relevant to his or her circumstances and needs.

The materials include:

1. A sample syllabus for a separate three–credit hour, one-semester pharmacology course. This syllabus was used by the author, with annual revisions, for about 15 years.
2. General observations and comments about teaching and learning pharmacology in relation to nursing.
3. General teaching strategies that aim to promote student interest in and attention to drug therapy. The importance of drug therapy cannot be overemphasized because there are few areas of nursing with similar potentials for helping or harming clients.
4. For each chapter of the text, this manual contains the following materials, any of which can be adapted to meet the needs of individual instructors:
   —major chapter topics
   —a quick reference guide to the text for objectives, displays (eg, boxes, figures, tables), and selected elements (eg, nursing process, principles of therapy, review and application exercises)
   —terms and concepts
   —a list of selected individual drugs, mainly prototypes and commonly used drugs
   —teaching strategies for classroom settings, cross-referenced to the transparencies to promote rapid retrieval and easier use. Most chapters include a new sub-section entitled "Collaborative activities for small groups."
   —teaching strategies for clinical settings, to facilitate application of drug knowledge in patient care
5. Discussion/solutions of case studies from the Study Guide are included to assist instructors in using the case studies for classroom discussion.

To fulfill the second purpose, testbank questions are provided for each chapter of the text (printed both in the manual and on disk, to facilitate use). These follow the NCLEX format.

Sample Course Syllabus

COURSE DESCRIPTION

Introduction to clinical drug therapy with emphasis on the knowledge and interventions needed to maximize therapeutic effects and prevent or minimize adverse effects of drugs. Major content areas include basic concepts of pharmacology, groups of therapeutic drugs, prototypes of drug groups, commonly prescribed individual drugs, drug effects on body tissues, human responses to drug therapy, applying nursing process in relation to prescribed drug therapy regimens, and principles of therapy in various circumstances and populations.

Faculty
Required Text(s)

COURSE OBJECTIVES

Upon completion of this course, the student should be able to:

1. Define/describe terms, concepts, and basic processes associated with drug therapy.
2. Use a systematic approach to studying drug therapy, with emphasis on therapeutic classifications and prototypical drugs.
3. Describe the pathophysiology of selected major conditions for which drug therapy is commonly used.
4. Describe characteristics of major drug groups and selected individual drugs in terms of the following:
   a. mechanism(s) of action
   b. indications for use
   c. contraindications to use
   d. expected therapeutic effects
   e. common or serious adverse effects
   f. accurate administration
   g. essential client teaching
5. Identify client-related and drug-related factors that influence drug effects.
6. Apply all steps of the nursing process in the care of clients receiving one or more therapeutic drugs.
7. Discuss principles of therapy with major drug groups in relation to drug selection, dosage, route, and use in special populations (eg, children, older adults, clients with impaired renal or hepatic function).
8. Discuss clinically significant drug–drug, drug–disease, and drug–nutrient interactions.
9. Discuss nursing process implications of administering or supervising drug therapy in the home setting.
10. Describe selected legal, ethical, and economic aspects of drug therapy.
11. Evaluate over-the-counter drugs for personal use or instruction of clients.

TOPICAL OUTLINE OF UNITS

I. Introduction to Drug Therapy
II. Drugs Affecting the Central Nervous System
III. Drugs Affecting the Autonomic Nervous System
IV. Drugs Affecting the Endocrine System
V. Nutrients, Fluids, and Electrolytes
VI. Drugs Used to Treat Infections
VII. Drugs Affecting Hematopoeisis and the Immune System
VIII. Drugs Affecting the Respiratory System
IX. Drugs Affecting the Cardiovascular System
X. Drugs Affecting the Digestive System
XI. Drugs Used in Special Conditions

TEACHING METHODS

Audiovisuals Case
Lecture/discussion
Required readings
Recommended readings

study analysis
Nursing process exercises
Small group activities
Written assignments

GRADING POLICIES

ATTENDANCE POLICIES

GENERAL OBSERVATIONS

1. Pharmacology is a basic science on a par with physiology, microbiology, chemistry, and so forth. Thus, similar study skills and time commitments are needed for learning and applying drug knowledge.
2. Students often say they feel overwhelmed by the number of drugs and amount of information they're expected to assimilate and apply to clinical practice. This seems to be a universal and growing problem as the number of commonly used drugs continues to expand.
3. The FDA approves many new drugs each year and has recently had several drugs taken off the market because of adverse effects. Thus, continued study and use of drug reference materials are required for this dynamic element of nursing practice.
4. One way to reduce the amount of drug-related material is to emphasize prototypical drugs. However, several important drug groups do not have clear-cut prototypes or the prototypical drug is no longer commonly used. In addition, instruction should not be limited to prototypes because such limitations do not adequately reflect the diversity and complexity of drug therapy in the clinical setting. Thus, each faculty group or individual instructor must decide which drugs to include or emphasize.

GENERAL TEACHING STRATEGIES

1. Provide students with a vocabulary list (terms and concepts) for each unit of instruction or assigned chapter in the pharmacology text. Terms and concepts may be studied independently, used as a basis for classroom questioning and discussion, or used for written assignments when considered complex or vital to understanding course content.
2. Provide students with a list of individual drugs for each unit of instruction or assigned chapter. For students, the drug list can limit the number of drugs to be studied (eg, a few from each chapter), delineate the drugs they are expected to know, and focus study efforts on important drugs. For instructors, the drug list can guide lectures, discussion topics, test items, and clinical teaching.
   a. List drugs by the generic name and a trade name. The generic name is especially important. Students need to become accustomed to both names, however, because drugs may be ordered by either one. Pharmacies and health care agencies vary in the trade names of drugs they dispense. Thus, the instructor may use trade names that are commonly used in students' clinical practice settings.
   b. The number of trade names in the text is necessarily limited because of space and other considerations. The instructor may suggest that students write in trade names of drugs they often encounter in clinical practice.
3. Provide students with learning objectives for each unit of instruction, group of drugs, or class period. These can be written by the instructor or assembled from chapter objectives in *Clinical Drug Therapy*, with objectives added or deleted as desired.
   a. Students can use the objectives to further their understanding of the instructor's expectations and to guide their study efforts.
   b. In the classroom, instructors can use the objectives as an outline for a lecture, as topics for class or small group discussions, or as topics for written homework assignments.

    c. In the clinical setting, instructors can consider the objectives in making students' client care assignments, use them for pre- or post-conference group discussions, or use them for questioning individual students about their clients' drug therapy regimens.

4. Use various approaches to focus students' attention at the beginning of class.
    a. Introduce the "topic of the day."
    b. Show transparencies of drug-related cartoons or comic strips.
    c. Start class with drug-related current events or "Drugs in the News" (often in newspapers). Ask students to contribute items.
    d. Describe the historical development of a drug or drug group. Useful information may include the date approved by the FDA, the impact on drug therapy, and whether the group is relatively dynamic or stable over time. For example, recent "dynamic" groups, to which several new drugs have been added, include fluoroquinolones, angiotensin II receptor antagonists, proton pump inhibitors, antiplatelet drugs, and "statins."

5. Use the review and application exercises at the end of each chapter of the text.
    a. Select one or more exercises to discuss in class.
    b. Have students individually write answers to one or more, in class or as a homework assignment.
    c. Assign students to small groups (3–5 students each) and have the groups discuss selected exercises and report to the whole class.

6. Make overhead transparencies of selected worksheets in the Study Guide and have the class complete the worksheets as an in-class exercise to stimulate and reinforce learning.

7. Discuss or ask students if they have questions about the interactive displays or the answers in the text.

8. Discuss critical thinking case study exercises (in several chapters of the student manual) as a class or in small groups. For the more complex exercises, an out-of-class written assignment may be more appropriate. Sample solutions are provided in the instructor's manual.

9. Have students complete a medication history on a client, friend, or family member who takes at least two prescription drugs daily.

10. Provide portions of nursing process information and have students use the information in planning nursing care.
    a. State a client's medical diagnosis and selected signs and symptoms, then ask students to identify laboratory or other diagnostic test data needed to evaluate the client's response to drug therapy.
    b. Provide a completed medication history, discuss other information, then have students state nursing diagnoses and goals.
    c. State one or more nursing diagnoses and have students state or write the interventions needed.
    d. Give students a list of diseases or signs and symptoms of a client and ask them to predict the type of drug or an individual drug that is likely to be prescribed.
    e. Give students a list of a client's drugs and ask them to predict the disease processes or signs and symptoms the client is probably experiencing.

11. Give students opportunities to learn and practice client teaching skills.
    a. Have each student write an individualized teaching plan about two prescription drugs, using his or her completed medication history.
    b. Have students look at teaching guidelines in relevant chapters of the text, then individualize instruction for a child, an older adult, or someone with renal failure.
    c. Provide a copy of an instruction sheet from a hospital or community pharmacy and ask the student to individualize it for an assigned client.

12. Have students "adopt-a-drug" related to course content and write a short paper in which the drug, its "family," clinical indications for use, adverse effects, client teaching implications, and other pertinent information are included. This is an opportunity for students to be creative and imaginative! Students may choose a drug with which they have had some personal experience, or drug names may be randomly drawn from a container. Prototypes or commonly used drugs are especially helpful.

13. Invite an occasional guest speaker, if feasible. Possibilities include a pharmacist from a hospital or community drugstore; a nutritionist; a nurse colleague with expertise in drug therapy with children, elderly, mentally ill, or other special populations; a nurse colleague with expertise in cardiovascular drugs, emergency or critical care drugs, or drug abuse and dependency; someone with diabetes and a family member; a member of a local senior citizen's group; or a member of a local support group for people with various disease processes or drug therapy regimens.

14. Most of the above strategies apply primarily to students in an introductory pharmacology course or a basic nursing program. For RNs with an associate degree who need a pharmacology course to complete a baccalaureate degree, their basic drug knowledge can be assessed and, if adequate, an independent study course can be designed to fill identified gaps while avoiding unnecessary repetition of basic information and maintaining student attendance. In addition, a student's areas of work or interest can be considered. One approach is described below:

    —Provide information about the course, including objectives, name of textbook, main topics and material covered, and so forth.

    —Administer the final exam for the course as a challenge exam. (Most students pass this exam, indicating they already have basic drug knowledge. The few students who fail the exam are unlikely candidates for independent study and need to attend the class.)

    —Analyze the test results to identify areas of incorrect answers (eg, cardiovascular or CNS drugs).

    —Confer with the student regarding test results, areas needing improved knowledge, and areas of work or special interest.

    —Have the student write learning objectives (about 6 to 10) and submit them for review.

    —Provide feedback and suggestions for finalizing the objectives.

    —Design learning activities such as textbook or journal reading assignments, written assignments (eg, analysis of case studies or patient care scenarios related to drug therapy, adopt-a-drug or a drug group as described above, answering review questions, listing contents of emergency box or cart where employed and stating reasons or circumstances for using each drug), viewing audiovisuals, and others. These need to be reasonable in terms of the time and effort required for completion.

    —In consultation with the student, write a contract for the grade the student wants. The contract specifies the work required for an A, B, or C.

    —Meet with the student two or three times during the semester to discuss and evaluate progress toward meeting objectives.

    —Award the earned grade at the end of the semester.

CONTENTS

INTRODUCTION TO DRUG THERAPY

CHAPTER 1

Introduction to Pharmacology

MAJOR TOPICS

- Sources and names of drugs
- Sources of drug information
- Federal drug laws and standards; scheduled drugs
- FDA drug-approval processes
- Cellular physiology and response to injury
- Chemical mediators of inflammation
- Actions of anti-inflammatory drugs

QUICK REFERENCE GUIDE TO TEXT

- Objectives, p. 3
- Interactive display, p. 6
- Box 1-1. Controlled substances, p. 5
- Box 1-2. Chemical mediators, p. 7
- Figure 1-1. Cell structures, p. 7
- Figure 1-2. Production of prostaglandins and leukotrienes; actions of anti-inflammatory drugs, p. 10
- Review and application exercises, p. 11

TERMS AND CONCEPTS

Biotechnology
Generic name
Inflammatory mediators
Leukotrienes
Prostaglandins

Prototype
Scheduled drugs
Systemic effects
Trade name

■ Teaching Strategies

CLASSROOM

1. Prepare and show a transparency of the 25 drugs most often prescribed for ambulatory clients (prepared from an annual list of the top 200 drugs dispensed in community pharmacies, usually published in the February or March issue of *American Druggist*). List the drugs by both generic and trade names. Ask students which they recognize, which they have given to clients, or which they have taken themselves. Many students recognize several drugs. This helps them realize that they already have some drug knowledge and are not starting from "ground zero."

2. Ask students to bring in a container of a prescription or OTC drug they have taken recently. List drug names on a transparency or marker board. For each one, add therapeutic classifications or major indications for use and whether it will be studied in the course. The purpose of this exercise is to create interest and motivation to learn about drug therapy, to emphasize that drug knowledge is relevant to personal lives as well as professional activities, and to emphasize that drug knowledge needs to be *used* (not just learned for a classroom test). The instructor may also use personal or family medications as examples.

3. Show copies of various sources of drug information (eg, textbooks, handbooks, *Physicians' Desk Reference, Drug Facts and Comparisons,* journal articles, and others) and discuss advantages and disadvantages of commonly used sources.

4. List a few reliable, authoritative web sites for obtaining drug information (eg, www.medscape.com; www.fda.gov). Discuss the pitfalls of obtaining information from nonauthoritative sites; this is an unregulated area in which anyone may establish a web site and disseminate whatever information they choose, whether accurate or not.

5. Provide a list of commonly used scheduled drugs. Ask students to designate the appropriate category of each drug and discuss nursing implications of administering the drug.

6. Show a transparency of Figure 1-1 (text, p. 7; transparency 1) to emphasize that body processes, including drug actions, occur at the cellular level.

7. Discuss the role of selected chemical mediators (Box 1-2, text, p. 8) in causing inflammation and the fact that many drugs act to decrease the activity of one or more of these substances.

8. Show a transparency of Figure 1-2 (text, p. 10; transparency 2) to provide an overview of anti-inflammatory drugs (eg, NSAIDs, corticosteroids, leukotriene inhibitors) that are commonly encountered in clinical practice.

CLINICAL LABORATORY

1. Have students identify scheduled drugs ordered for assigned clients.

2. Have each student select at least 2 drugs prescribed for an assigned client and consult a drug reference or make drug cards with important information. Course objective 4 (p. vi) can be used as an outline or format for content to be included. Encourage students to use their own words rather than copying the information. The mental processing required to restate the information aids learning and retention.

3. Have students look at a physician's order sheet for an assigned client and indicate whether drug names are generic or trade names.

4. Review with students the agency's policies related to scheduled drugs.

5. In a hospital setting, have one or more students list the scheduled drugs (from the medication administration record [MAR]) of several or all clients. This exercise helps students get a feel for the extent of use in that unit and which individual drugs are more commonly used.

6. Ask students to identify signs and symptoms of inflammation observed in assigned clients, if any.

7. Ask students to state examples of drugs used for systemic effects and drugs used for local effects.

CHAPTER 2

Basic Concepts and Processes

MAJOR TOPICS

- Mechanisms of drug movement—passive diffusion, facilitated diffusion, active transport

- Pharmacokinetics—absorption, distribution, biotransformation, excretion

- Pathologic processes (eg, cardiovascular, renal, hepatic diseases) that influence drug pharmacokinetics

- Pharmacodynamics—receptor theory of drug action at the cellular level

- Drug-related variables that affect drug actions

- Client-related variables that affect drug actions

- Adverse drug reactions

QUICK REFERENCE GUIDE TO TEXT

- Objectives, p. 12

- Interactive displays, pp. 12, 15, and 18

- Figure 2-1. Drug binding to serum albumin, p. 14

- Figure 2-2. Drug binding to receptors on cell membranes, p. 15

- Table 2-1. Effects of pathologic conditions on drug pharmacokinetics, p. 21

- Review and application exercises, p. 24

TERMS AND CONCEPTS

Agonist
Agranulocytosis
Antagonist
Carcinogenicity
Displacement
Enzyme induction
Enzyme inhibition
Hepatotoxicity
Hypersensitivity

Leukopenia
Nephrotoxicity
Passive diffusion
Pharmacodynamics
Pharmacokinetics—absorption, distribution, biotransformation, excretion
Protein binding

Receptor theory of drug action
Teratogenicity

Tolerance and cross-tolerance

■ Teaching Strategies

Classroom

1. Lecture/discussion of pharmacokinetic processes and influencing factors:
   a. Define absorption and describe factors that increase or decrease absorption of an oral tablet or capsule (eg, rate of dissolution in gastric fluids, GI tract motility, presence of other drugs or foods in the GI tract, blood flow to the GI tract).
   b. Define distribution. Discuss the need for adequate cardiovascular function to maintain blood flow to body tissues. Show a transparency of Figure 2-1 (text, p. 14; transparency 3) and discuss the importance of adequate plasma proteins (eg, serum albumin) to bind drug molecules. Emphasize that only free or unbound drug molecules can leave the bloodstream and act on body tissues.
   c. Define metabolism and biotransformation. Discuss the importance of adequate blood flow to the liver and factors that induce or inhibit drug-metabolizing enzymes in the liver.
   d. Define excretion and discuss the importance of kidney function in relation to eliminating drug molecules and metabolites from the body.
   e. Select a disorder of a body system in Table 2-1 and discuss how that disorder affects one or more pharmacokinetic processes. Renal and hepatic disorders are especially important in drug metabolism and excretion.

2. Lecture/discussion of the receptor theory of drug action:
   a. Describe characteristics of receptors.
   b. Show a transparency of Figure 2-2 (text, p. 15; transparency 4).

c. Emphasize that many drugs are similar to naturally occurring body substances.

3. Discuss selected variables that affect drug action (eg, drug dosage, client's weight and health status).

4. Emphasize the need to actively assess clients for adverse drug reactions (ADRs) because ADRs may cause virtually any sign or symptom.

5. Show a transparency of major body systems affected by ADRs and ask students how they would recognize the ADRs (ie, specific signs and symptoms) (transparency 5).

6. Show a transparency of ways to monitor clients for ADRs (transparency 6).

7. State a serum albumin level; ask whether a client with this level is at increased risk for ADRs. Ask students to state rationales for their answers.

Clinical Laboratory

1. Ask students to assess assigned clients for gastrointestinal, cardiovascular, hepatic, or renal disorders that could interfere with absorption, distribution, metabolism, or excretion of drugs.

2. Ask students to assess clients for at least one specific ADR that may occur with the client's prescribed drug therapy regimen.

3. Ask students to record laboratory reports (eg, serum albumin, blood urea nitrogen, serum creatinine, AST, ALT), when available for an assigned client, and evaluate the client's risk for ADRs or drug-drug interactions.

CHAPTER 3

Administering Medications

MAJOR TOPICS

- Five rights of drug administration
- Medication orders/prescriptions
- Drug preparations and dosage forms
- Calculating drug dosages
- Routes of administration
- General techniques of drug administration

QUICK REFERENCE GUIDE TO TEXT

- Objectives, p. 26
- Interactive displays, pp. 27 and 33
- Table 3-1. Common abbreviations, p. 28
- Table 3-2. Equivalents, p. 29
- Figures 3-1 through 3-5. Injection sites, pp. 32 and 33
- Nursing process, p. 33
- Review and application exercises, p. 40

TERMS AND CONCEPTS

Enteric-coated   Sustained-release
Milliequivalents   Topical
Parenteral   Transdermal

■ Teaching Strategies

CLASSROOM

1. List and discuss advantages and disadvantages of various routes of drug administration.

2. If not previously covered elsewhere, show equipment (eg, oral and parenteral unit-dose medications, needles, and syringes) and discuss criteria for selecting them.

3. Ask which specific equipment/site/technique would be appropriate for
   a. An SC injection.
   b. An IM injection for an 8-month-old child, an obese adult, and a debilitated adult.
   c. Administering a liquid and a pill via a nasogastric tube.

4. Discuss the types of drugs often given PRN (eg, analgesics, antiemetics) and the criteria the nurse may use to guide decision-making about administration of PRN medications.

5. Discuss possible approaches to an adult client who refuses an important medication.

6. Discuss possible interventions when assessment of a client's condition seems to contraindicate a particular drug or a particular dose of a drug.

7. Discuss possible replies and actions when a client questions the number or types of medications being offered.

8. Discuss possible interventions when a student realizes he or she has given a medication to the wrong patient or made a medication error in relation to any of the 5 rights.

9. Discuss possible interventions when a student discovers that someone else has made a medication error in relation to any of the 5 rights.

10. Discuss possible interventions when a nurse or a student suspects a coworker of drug abuse.

11. Discuss safety factors related to drug administration to children and elderly adults, and in hospital and home settings.

CLINICAL LABORATORY

1. Discuss a specific institution's policies and procedures regarding drug administration and recording.

2. In a hospital or long-term care facility, have students administer medications to their assigned clients, including alternative routes (eg, NG tube, injection, inhalation, topically to skin).

3. Have students analyze assigned clients' medications for
   a. Drugs given for systemic effects.
   b. Drugs given for local effects.
   c. Nonoral dosage forms and routes of administration.
   d. Tablets or capsules that should not be crushed.
   e. Drugs that may be left at the bedside.
   f. Drugs that may be self-administered by the client.
   g. Type, frequency of administration, reason for use, and effects of PRN drugs.
   h. Questions a client might ask about a drug and appropriate ways to answer them.

4. In an outpatient setting, have students ask clients about how they self-administer their medications and have students evaluate methods in relation to safe administration practices (for medications in general and for specific drugs the client is taking).

CHAPTER 4

Nursing Process in Drug Therapy

MAJOR TOPICS

- Legal responsibilities of the nurse
- Applying the nursing process in drug therapy: assessment; nursing diagnoses; planning/goals; interventions (including teaching); and evaluation.
- General principles of drug therapy: goals; benefits versus risks; drug selection; and individualization in special populations (ie, children, older adults, clients with impaired renal or hepatic function, and clients who are critically ill).

QUICK REFERENCE GUIDE TO TEXT

- Objectives, p. 41
- Interactive displays, pp. 41 and 52
- Nursing process, pp. 43 and 58
- Box 4-1. Medication history, p. 44
- Client teaching guidelines: Prescription drugs, p. 46
- Client teaching guidelines: Over-the-counter drugs, p. 47
- General principles of drug therapy, p. 50
- Table 4-1. Children: Physiologic characteristics and pharmacokinetic consequences, p. 51
- Figure 4-1. Body surface nomogram, p. 52
- Table 4-2. Older adults: Physiologic characteristics and pharmacokinetic consequences, p. 54
- Review and application exercises, p. 59

TERMS AND CONCEPTS

Drug classification	Maintenance doses
Chronologic age	Physiologic age
Clinical pathways	Quality of life
Loading doses	

■ Teaching Strategies

CLASSROOM

1. Emphasize that students already know the steps of the nursing process; now they need to apply those steps in drug therapy.

2. Show a transparency of the medication history (Box 4-1, text, p. 44; transparency 7) and discuss the rationale for obtaining the designated information. Emphasize that the information can readily be incorporated into any assessment tool and that a separate medication history is not required.

3. Ask students to identify additional sources of drug-related information, including various textbooks and a client's medical records.

4. Demonstrate ways to analyze assessment data to determine the client's nursing care needs related to drug therapy (eg, implications related to the client's age and medical diagnoses as well as the prescribed drugs).

5. Ask students to identify laboratory tests that help to assess a client's response to drug therapy (therapeutic or adverse).

6. Emphasize that students already know principles of teaching/learning; now they need to apply the principles in relation to drug therapy. They also need to consider the client's education and reading level.

7. Discuss information a client usually needs about a newly prescribed drug and resources and methodologies for providing this information.

8. For a client who has been taking a drug for a while, discuss assessment of learning needs in relation to the drug. Ask students to state specific questions that can be used to assess a client's knowledge and medication-taking behavior.

Emphasize that long-term use of a drug does not indicate adequate knowledge or correct use.

9. For a client who has been started on a new drug while hospitalized, discuss factors to be considered in discharge teaching about the drug. How does the new drug fit with the client's other drugs (if any)? Are there activity or dietary restrictions needed with the new drug? What if the patient is a child or an elderly adult?

10. Provide a client care situation and ask students to write a teaching plan for at least 2 medications. Some guidelines are provided in the Teaching Plan for Medications section.

11. Provide a copy of a drug information sheet dispensed with an outpatient prescription drug. Have students critique it for usefulness for an individual patient (actual or hypothetical) and individualize it for that patient.

12. Show one or more clinical pathways (from an agency or a textbook) to demonstrate the relationship of drug therapy to other elements.

13. Discuss costs of medications. Costs can be obtained from journal articles (eg, *Medical Letter on Drugs and Therapeutics*), or the instructor and students can share their experiences and personal purchases.

COLLABORATIVE ACTIVITIES FOR SMALL GROUPS

1. Provide assessment information and a list of drugs ordered for a client; assign small groups to write a nursing care plan (nursing diagnoses, goals, interventions, evaluation criteria).

2. Divide the class into small groups and name a commonly used drug (one likely to be familiar to some students). Assign half of the groups to discuss item 8 in the Classroom section and half to discuss item 9. Have one or two groups from each half to share their findings with the whole class.

3. Provide a client care situation and ask groups to write a teaching plan for at least two medications. Some guidelines are provided in the Teaching Plan for Medications section.

4. Provide a copy of or information from an OTC drug label and have students critique it for use by themselves or by most patients.

CLINICAL LABORATORY

1. For an assigned client, have students complete a medication history, obtain additional assessment

data from the client's medical records, analyze data with the help of appropriate references and textbooks, and write a nursing care plan that reflects the client's needs related to drug therapy.

2. Have students do initial and discharge teaching of clients when the opportunity arises.

3. Given 2 patients receiving the same drug, ask students to compare and contrast assessment data (including whether the drug is newly prescribed or long-term) in relation to important information about the drug and to compare and contrast the teaching/learning needs of the 2 clients. This exercise helps reinforce the principle that all drug therapy should be individualized.

4. For clients at home, have students review the drugs being taken and provide clients an opportunity to ask questions, state concerns, and identify any difficulties they have encountered with the medications.

TEACHING PLAN FOR MEDICATIONS

1. For a "general" teaching plan related to a particular drug, include information that is likely to be helpful to most people for whom the drug is prescribed.

2. For a specific client, consider client-related factors (eg, age, medical diagnosis, laboratory and other diagnostic test reports, nursing database, medication history) and drug-related information (eg, type of drug, indications for use, adverse effects) to assess the client's learning needs about a particular drug. More specifically, try to determine the following:
   a. What does the client already know?
   b. What does the client need to know?
   c. What does the client want to know?

3. Write specific, measurable, attainable objectives (eg, use action verbs such as *list*, *write*, *verbalize*, and *state* rather than *know* or *understand*).

4. List content to be covered. (With a newly prescribed drug, most of the information listed here is needed. With a drug the client has been taking for a while, specific content is determined by the client's knowledge about the drug and the nurse's assessment data about the client's compliance, therapeutic and adverse responses, and other individualized information.)
   a. Name of drug.
   b. Reason for use (what it will do for the client in terms of relieving symptoms, preventing problems, and so on).
   c. Prescribing information (eg, dose, frequency of administration).

d. Adverse effects to be reported.

e. Preparation or storage instructions, if indicated.

5. List methods of instruction, including verbal, written (self or booklets), and audiovisual aids.

6. To evaluate teaching, state criteria indicating whether objective was met or not met.

7. Use four columns, with the following headings: Objectives, Content, Methods of Instruction, and Evaluation.

■ Critical Thinking Case Study

M. weighs 44 lb or 20 kg.

1. If the recommended dosage range of phenobarbital is 4–6 mg/kg/day, then the maximum daily dose should be 120 mg/day.

2. If the medication is administered in 3 equal doses, M. should receive 40 mg per dose.

3. Phenobarbital comes in a formulation of 15 mg/mL. You should administer 2.66 mL or 2.7 mL.

4. The minimum dose of Dilantin is 80 mg/day or 40 mg bid.

5. The maximum dose of Dilantin is 140 mg/day or 70 mg bid.

6. If you are administering 70 mg per dose, you would give 1.4 mL.

7. The medication could be administered in the abdomen, thigh, arm.

8. The maximum dose for M. should be 4 mg. The order exceeds the maximum dose; therefore the nurse should speak with the physician.

DRUGS AFFECTING THE CENTRAL NERVOUS SYSTEM

CHAPTER 5

Physiology of the Central Nervous System

MAJOR TOPICS

- Neurotransmitters, synapses, receptors
- Neurotransmission systems—cholinergic, dopaminergic, GABA-ergic, noradrenergic, serotonergic
- Major CNS structures and their functions
- Drugs affecting the CNS: depressants and stimulants

QUICK REFERENCE GUIDE TO TEXT

- Objectives, p. 63
- Figure 5-1. Neurotransmission, p. 64
- Review and application exercises, p. 70

TERMS AND CONCEPTS

Acetylcholine	Norepinephrine
Dopamine	Receptors
Neuron	Serotonin
Neurotransmission systems	Synapse

■ Teaching Strategies

CLASSROOM

1. Assign the chapter to be read before discussion of antianxiety, antipsychotic, and antidepressant medications. Information about neurotransmitters, receptors, and so on is essential to understanding the clinical effects of these drugs.

2. Discuss CNS neurotransmission systems.

3. Show a transparency of Figure 5-1 (text, p. 64; transparency 8).

4. Discuss common disorders associated with deficiency or excess of particular neurotransmitters.

5. Discuss drug actions that mimic or block actions of naturally occurring neurotransmitters.

6. Discuss review and application exercises 7 and 8 (text, p. 70).

CLINICAL LABORATORY

1. Have students assess each assigned client in terms of level of consciousness and overt mental health status.

2. For assigned clients, ask students to identify those with either disease processes or drug therapy regimens associated with altered neurotransmitter functions.

CHAPTER 6

Opioid Analgesics and Opioid Antagonists

MAJOR TOPICS

- Pain
- Description of opioid analgesics
- Classifications and individual drugs
- Nursing process in relation to pain assessment and management
- Principles of therapy, including use in special populations and management of drug overdose or withdrawal

QUICK REFERENCE GUIDE TO TEXT

- Objectives, p. 71
- Interactive displays, pp. 71 and 79
- Table 6-1. Opioid receptors, p. 75
- Nursing process, pp. 78 and 86
- Client teaching guidelines: Opioid (narcotic) analgesics, p. 80
- Principles of therapy, p. 80
- Review and application exercises, p. 89

TERMS AND CONCEPTS

Analgesia
Endogenous analgesia system
Endorphins
Equianalgesia
Nociceptors

Opioid receptors
Pain
Patient-controlled
  analgesia

DRUG LIST

- Codeine
- Meperidine (Demerol)
- Morphine sulfate
- Naloxone (Narcan)
- Acetaminophen with codeine (eg, Tylenol No. 3)
- Hydrocodone/acetaminophen (eg, Hydrocet, Lorcet, Lortab, Vicodin)
- Oxycodone/acetaminophen (eg, Percocet, Roxicet, Tylox)

■ Teaching Strategies

CLASSROOM

1. Compare and contrast acute pain and chronic pain.

2. Discuss nursing assessment of pain, including whether pain is objective (a sign) or subjective (a symptom).

3. Describe or demonstrate various pain assessment scales and tools.

4. Discuss interventions to prevent pain and nonpharmacologic methods of relieving pain.

5. Lecture/discussion about morphine as the prototype opioid analgesic in terms of mechanism of action, indications for use, therapeutic effects, common or serious adverse effects, accurate administration, and essential client/family teaching.

6. Ask students about factors the nurse should consider in deciding whether to give or not give a PRN opioid analgesic. Write factors on a transparency or marker board. Put an asterisk or checkmark by those factors with a high degree of consensus; discuss factors with low consensus further.

7. Discuss the nursing care of a client receiving an intravenous analgesic (by continuous infusion or PCA pump) or epidural opioid analgesic.

8. Ask students to share their experiences with pain and their methods of relieving pain.

9. Outline treatment measures for opioid overdose, including indications for use and expected effects of an opioid antagonist.

10. Discuss pain management as a component of perioperative care.

11. Compare and contrast opioid and nonopioid analgesics in terms of effectiveness and adverse effects.

12. Discuss the rationale for combining opioid and nonopioid analgesics.

13. Compare the nursing implications of administering strong parenteral opioids and oral opioid/nonopioid combination drugs.

14. Ask students to compare and contrast options for pain management in a client with acute pain (eg, traumatic injury or 1–2 days after major surgery) and in a client with chronic cancer pain. Factors may include individual drugs, dosages, routes and frequencies of administration, and specific signs and symptoms of adverse drug effects. The instructor may list the options identified by students and add others to ensure that significant points are included.

15. For a home care client, discuss ways to increase the safety of opioid analgesic administration.

COLLABORATIVE ACTIVITIES FOR SMALL GROUPS

1. Assign groups to discuss the client scenario (text, p. 71) and list assessment data and important elements of client/family teaching.

2. Choose one or more special populations (eg, children, older adults, people with cancer, perioperative status, renal or hepatic impairment) and have 1 or more groups list needed assessment data and interventions.

3. Assign groups to complete the Critical Thinking Case Study (study guide, p. 20) over about 10 minutes. Then, ask 2 or 3 groups to report their findings. Next, ask other students whether they agree with the groups' findings or have other additions or suggestions. The instructor can list important points on a marker board or overhead transparency, if desired.

CLINICAL LABORATORY

1. When making assignments, ask each student assigned to a client receiving an opioid analgesic to list the drug, dose, route and frequency of administration, and client's responses. During postconference discussions, ask affected students to share their information with other students. Encourage students to discuss, question, and state possible reasons for using a particular drug, dose, or route in a particular client. In addition, ask students whether they think a patient's pain is being managed effectively. If not, ask them to identify other strategies or options that might be more effective.

2. For a client receiving an opioid analgesic, have a student assess the level of consciousness, respiratory status, and other safety factors and verbalize at least 1 nursing diagnosis relevant to the drug therapy.

3. Assign a student to assess a client's need for a pain medication, administer an opioid analgesic, and evaluate the client's response about 30 minutes after drug administration.

4. Ask a patient with a PCA pump or epidural opioid analgesic for permission to show the device to students who have not previously seen it. Include the patient in any demonstration or discussion that occurs at the bedside. Interview the client regarding effectiveness of the method in managing pain and any difficulties experienced with it.

5. Have students list the opioid/nonopioid analgesics (eg, generic and trade names and amounts of each ingredient) that are commonly used in the clinical agency.

6. Discuss morphine dosage forms and dosage ranges for various clinical uses.

■ Critical Thinking Case Study

1. "It is necessary to begin to decrease your pain medication so that you do not become dependent on it. We will wean you gradually off the medication while we increase your activity, and that should control your pain."

2. Constipation is a common adverse effect of administration of narcotic analgesics. Daily documentation of bowel patterns, increased mobility, roughage, and fluid intake should help to minimize constipation.

3. You should start by finding out the location and extent of pain that M.G. was experiencing. You need to document the teaching that you did with M.G. in the morning. Your plan for weaning M.G. off the pain medication needs to be discussed with the other staff members and included in the plan of care. M.G. also needs additional teaching.

CHAPTER 7

Analgesic–Antipyretic–Anti-inflammatory and Related Drugs

MAJOR TOPICS

- Prostaglandins and their effects
- Characteristics of fever, pain, inflammation, gout, and migraine
- Characteristics of aspirin and NSAIDs, including COX-2 inhibitors
- Use of "triptan" drugs in treating migraine
- Nursing process and principles of therapy related to clients with fever, pain, inflammation, gout, and migraine
- Management of acetaminophen overdose

QUICK REFERENCE GUIDE TO TEXT

- Objectives, p. 90
- Interactive displays, pp. 90 and 103
- Table 7-1. Prostaglandins and their effects, p. 91
- Figure 7-1. Formation of prostaglandins and actions of anti-inflammatory drugs, p. 92
- Table 7-2. Clinical indications for analgesic–antipyretic–anti-inflammatory drugs, pp. 94
- Nursing process, pp. 98 and 105
- Client teaching guidelines: Acetaminophen, aspirin, and other NSAIDs, p. 99
- Client teaching guidelines: Drugs for migraine, p. 101
- Principles of therapy, p. 100
- Review and application exercises, p. 109

TERMS AND CONCEPTS

Antipyretic

Arachidonic acid

Cyclooxygenase

Prostaglandins

DRUG LIST

- Acetaminophen (Tylenol, others)
- Acetylcysteine (Mucomyst)
- Aspirin
- Celecoxib (Celebrex)
- Ibuprofen (Motrin, Advil, others)
- Naproxen (Naprosyn, Aleve)
- Rofecoxib (Vioxx)
- Sumatriptan (Imitrex)

■ Teaching Strategies

CLASSROOM

1. Show a transparency of Table 7-1 (text, p. 91; transparency 9) and discuss antiprostaglandin effects of aspirin and related drugs.

2. Ask about students' experiences with aspirin, acetaminophen, and ibuprofen (eg, personal preference and why, conditions drugs were used for, what kind of results were obtained, and whether they used generic or trade formulations).

3. Compare similarities and differences of selected drugs in terms of clinical indications for use (Table 7-2, text, p. 94; transparency 11).

4. Ask students to compare and contrast aspirin, acetaminophen, ibuprofen, and celecoxib in terms of indications for use and adverse effects.

5. Show a transparency of Figure 7-1 (text, p. 92; transparency 10) to illustrate and differentiate the actions of traditional NSAIDs and COX-2 inhibitors.

6. Describe the main advantage of COX-2 inhibitors over traditional NSAIDs.

7. Given a client with a nursing diagnosis of Risk for Injury related to aspirin or NSAID-induced gastric ulceration and gastrointestinal bleeding, have students identify or write nursing interventions to reduce risk.

8. Discuss major elements of treating overdoses of aspirin, other NSAIDs, and acetaminophen.

COLLABORATIVE ACTIVITIES FOR SMALL GROUPS

1. Assign groups to discuss review and application exercises 4, 5, and 6 (text, p. 109) regarding drug selection for a child, a middle-aged adult, and an elderly adult.

2. Assign groups to complete the Critical Thinking Case Study (study guide, p. 23) then discuss as a class.

3. Ask groups to prepare a teaching plan for a client taking one of the following drugs at home: an anti-inflammatory dose of ibuprofen, an antiplatelet dose of aspirin, or a "triptan" drug for migraine.

CLINICAL LABORATORY

1. For clients receiving aspirin or an NSAID, have students assess for knowledge about safe use and risk for adverse effects.

2. For clients receiving aspirin or an NSAID, have students question them about the occurrence of adverse drug effects.

3. For clients receiving aspirin or an NSAID, have students prepare a teaching plan and include OTC sources of the same or a similar drug.

4. Given a client who takes OTC preparations of aspirin, acetaminophen, or ibuprofen, have students instruct the client to read labels and follow instructions to ensure optimal therapeutic effects and minimize adverse effects.

5. During home visits, have students assess age, health status, and use of prescription or OTC NSAIDs for all members of the household. Intervene when indicated.

■ Critical Thinking Case Study

1. Uncommon but potential adverse effects related to Clinoril include gastrointestinal ulceration, hemolytic anemia, confusion, depression, and psychosis. The physician should be made aware of Mrs. J.'s past history of anemia and psychosis.

2. The periodic assessment would include a complete blood count to assess for anemia and bone marrow depression.

3. The nurse should teach Mrs. J. to avoid OTC medications, to avoid overuse of medications, and to use other measures instead of or along with drug therapy (eg, moist heat, massage, acupuncture).

4. Ketorolac is effective for the treatment of severe pain associated with arthritis and reportedly causes less gastric irritation than sulindac does. This medication can also be given by injection and is reportedly comparable to morphine in its analgesic effectiveness. Ketorolac is recommended for short-term use. For long-term use, etodolac (Lodine) would be appropriate.

CHAPTER 8

Antianxiety and Sedative-Hypnotic Drugs

MAJOR TOPICS

- Anxiety
- Benzodiazepines
- Benzodiazepine receptors
- Gamma-aminobutyric acid (GABA) as an inhibitory neurotransmitter
- Sleep patterns and disorders
- Management of benzodiazepine toxicity

QUICK REFERENCE GUIDE TO TEXT

- Objectives, p. 110
- Interactive displays, pp. 110 and 120
- Table 8-1. Barbiturates, p. 113
- Table 8-2. Benzodiazepines, p. 114
- Table 8-3. Miscellaneous drugs, p. 116
- Nursing process, pp. 117 and 124
- Client teaching guidelines: Antianxiety and sedative-hypnotic drugs, p. 119
- Principles of therapy, p. 120
- Review and application exercises, p. 128

TERMS AND CONCEPTS

Anxiety
Anxiolytic
Benzodiazepine-GABA receptor complex
Insomnia

DRUG LIST

- Alprazolam (Xanax)
- Buspirone (BuSpar)
- Diazepam (Valium)
- Flumazenil (Romazicon)
- Lorazepam (Ativan)
- Temazepam (Restoril)

■ Teaching Strategies

CLASSROOM

1. Discuss various terms a client might use to describe anxiety.
2. Discuss appearances and behaviors that might indicate anxiety.
3. Ask students how they feel when anxious and what they do to relieve anxiety.
4. Ask students if they think sleep is necessary for health.
5. Ask students to describe how they feel when they have had enough sleep, compared with the way they feel when sleep deprived.
6. Discuss consequences or potential hazards of sleep deprivation.
7. List "sleep hygiene" factors that anyone can use to develop healthful sleep habits.
8. Give students about 5 minutes to write a list of nonpharmacologic interventions to decrease anxiety and insomnia, then discuss as a group.
9. Discuss the benefits of nonpharmacologic versus pharmacologic treatment of anxiety.
10. Show a transparency of antianxiety benzodiazepines (transparency 12).
11. Show a transparency of hypnotic benzodiazepines (transparency 13).

12. Discuss client behaviors and verbal statements that may indicate a likelihood of compliance or abuse with prescribed hypnotic drugs.

13. Discuss the importance of teaching clients not to stop a benzodiazepine abruptly if it has been taken for longer than a few days.

COLLABORATIVE ACTIVITIES FOR SMALL GROUPS

1. Ask students to discuss one or more of review and application exercises 4, 8, 11, and 12 (text, p. 128); then ask selected groups to report their findings to the class as a whole.

2. For about 10 minutes, have half of the groups list all the circumstances they can think of in which an antianxiety drug or sleeping pill would be indicated for a client; assign the other half to list circumstances or clients for whom the drugs should generally not be given. Ask selected groups to report and provide rationales for their inclusions or exclusions.

3. Ask one or more groups to imagine working in a hospital emergency room when someone is admitted with a possible overdose of Valium. Ask students to list the needed assessment data and the expected sequence of events in treatment.

CLINICAL LABORATORY

1. When observing behaviors that may indicate anxiety, interview the client (if possible) to validate feelings of anxiety. The instructor or a student may conduct the interview.

2. For an outpatient who takes an antianxiety or sedative-hypnotic drug, ask a student to teach safety measures, including listing other drugs that increase sedative effects.

3. For a client receiving an antianxiety or sedative-hypnotic drug, identify behaviors or verbal statements that may indicate a risk of overuse or abuse of the drug.

4. For a client with a nursing diagnosis of Sleep Pattern Disturbance: Insomnia, assign a student to assess for lifestyle and environmental etiologic factors and list interventions appropriate to the client and the assessment data.

5. For a client with a nursing diagnosis of Knowledge Deficit with regard to nondrug measures for relieving stress and anxiety, have a student lead a postconference group discussion about appropriate interventions.

6. For a hospitalized client with a nursing diagnosis of Risk for Injury related to sedation and other adverse effects, have a student lead a postconference group discussion about interventions to protect the client.

7. In any clinical setting, have a student determine the location of (or the procedure for obtaining) flumazenil and report to the entire clinical group.

CHAPTER 9

Antipsychotic Drugs

MAJOR TOPICS

- Psychosis
- Schizophrenia
- Neurotransmission systems in psychosis
- Typical and atypical antipsychotic drugs

QUICK REFERENCE GUIDE TO TEXT

- Objectives, p. 129
- Interactive displays, pp. 129, 137, and 139
- Figure 9-1. Action of antipsychotic drugs, p. 131
- Nursing process, pp. 137 and 143
- Client teaching guidelines: Antipsychotic drugs, p. 138
- Principles of therapy, p. 139
- Review and application exercises, p. 148

TERMS AND CONCEPTS

Akathisia	Dystonia
Chemoreceptor trigger zone (CTZ)	Hallucinations
	Parkinsonism
Delusions	Photosensitivity
Dopamine	Tardive dyskinesia

DRUG LIST

- Chlorpromazine (Thorazine)
- Haloperidol (Haldol)
- Olanzapine (Zyprexa)
- Risperidone (Risperdal)

■ Teaching Strategies

CLASSROOM

1. Ask students what verbal and nonverbal behaviors would make them suspect psychosis.

2. Discuss phenothiazines and related drugs as the prototypical drugs in this category.

3. Differentiate older drugs from the newer, atypical agents.

4. Show a transparency of Figure 9-1 (text, p. 131; transparency 14) to demonstrate a postulated mechanism of drug action.

5. Discuss possible approaches to promote compliance with a prescribed antipsychotic drug therapy regimen.

6. For outpatients, discuss the importance of teaching a family member or caregiver about drug therapy.

7. Discuss specific appearances and behaviors that may indicate adverse effects of antipsychotic drugs, and list interventions for minimizing each adverse effect.

8. Discuss the client/family situation described in the display (text, p. 129).

COLLABORATIVE ACTIVITIES FOR SMALL GROUPS

1. Assign one or more groups to discuss selected review and application exercises (eg, numbers 7, 9, and 11, text, p. 148) and share findings with the entire class.

2. For clients in hospitals or long-term care facilities who become agitated, noisy, and disruptive, assign groups to discuss the ethical issue of applying "chemical restraints" in the form of sedating antipsychotic drugs.

3. Assign groups to discuss the Critical Thinking Case Study (study guide, p. 30) and report their findings to the class.

CLINICAL LABORATORY

1. For a client receiving a traditional antipsychotic drug, ask a student to assess for sedation, hypotension, anticholinergic effects, and extrapyramidal effects and verbally report assessment data to the instructor.

2. For a client with a nursing diagnosis of Impaired Physical Mobility related to sedation, ask the clinical group to list nursing interventions to increase client safety and decrease risks of injury.

3. For a client who has taken a phenothiazine or related antipsychotic drug for several years, have a student use the Abnormal Involuntary Movement Scale (AIMS) to assess for tardive dyskinesia.

4. For a client receiving haloperidol, olanzapine, quetiapine, or risperidone, discuss appearances or behaviors that may indicate adverse drug reactions.

■ Critical Thinking Case Study

1. Antipsychotic medications are contraindicated for persons with liver damage, coronary artery disease, cerebral vascular disease, parkinsonism, bone marrow depression, severe hypotension or hypertension, coma, or severely depressed state.

2. His symptoms could be those of acute psychosis. Administer an intramuscular injection of 1.25 mg initially, then gradually increase the dose to 2.5–10 mg daily given in 3 to 4 divided doses.

3. Prolixin acts within hours to decrease manifestations of hyperarousal. It can be administered in various forms, including an elixir that can be mixed with a variety of noncaffeinated beverages.

4. It may take several weeks or months of drug therapy and counseling to eliminate thought disorders and increase socialization.

5. An adverse effect associated with the use of Prolixin is transient, mild drowsiness initially. The drowsiness should improve. His dosage can be adjusted if this remains a problem.

6. "I will have the physician evaluate your father. There are a variety of things that this could be related to."

7. The following areas should be addressed before discharge: perform regular blood studies to evaluate creatinine, BUN, and WBCs; encourage fluids to avoid dehydration; assess for tardive dyskinesias; and tell the client, "Do not discontinue medication if there are problems; instead, contact your physician."

CHAPTER 10

● Antidepressants

MAJOR TOPICS

- Major depression
- Types of antidepressant drugs
- Neurotransmission systems in major depression
- Lithium therapy
- Management of drug toxicity/overdose

QUICK REFERENCE GUIDE TO TEXT

- Objectives, p. 150
- Interactive displays, pp. 150 and 159
- Table 10-1. Foods and drugs to be avoided during therapy with monoamine oxidase inhibitor drugs, p. 153
- Table 10-2. Antidepressant drugs, p. 155
- Nursing process, pp. 157 and 164
- Client teaching guidelines: Antidepressants and lithium, p. 158
- Principles of therapy, p. 159
- Review and application exercises, p. 167

TERMS AND CONCEPTS

Bipolar disorder	Serotonin
Mania and hypomania	Unipolar disorder
Monoamine oxidase	

DRUG LIST

- Amitriptyline (Elavil)
- Fluoxetine (Prozac)
- Lithium (Eskalith, others)
- Mirtazapine (Remeron)
- Sertraline (Zoloft)

■ Teaching Strategies

CLASSROOM

1. Try to focus students' attention by asking for their opinions/observations about the prevalence of depression among college students and other young adults. (Suicide is a leading cause of death among adolescents and young adults.)

2. Ask students what appearances and behaviors would make them think a client is depressed.

3. Ask students about ways to distinguish between temporary sadness that does not require drug therapy and major depression, which often does require drug therapy.

4. Show a transparency of the major groups of antidepressants (transparency 15).

5. Discuss TCAs as the prototypes and SSRIs as the most commonly used drugs.

6. Compare TCAs and SSRIs in terms of adverse drug effects.

7. Have students write brief descriptions of the mechanism of action for major types of antidepressants.

8. Discuss the importance of teaching clients that optimal therapeutic effects may not occur until they have been taking the drug for 2–3 weeks.

9. Discuss laboratory monitoring of clients taking lithium.

10. Discuss the rationale for adequate sodium intake during lithium therapy.

11. Identify community resources (both on and off campus) for depressed persons.

COLLABORATIVE ACTIVITIES FOR SMALL GROUPS

1. Assign groups to list and discuss assessment data and potentially helpful interventions for a depressed client, friend, or family member.

2. Ask each group to imagine a friend who seems depressed and possibly suicidal. Then, ask students to share how they might feel and behave in such a circumstance.

3. Assign about half the groups to discuss the client care scenario (text, p. 150) and the other half to discuss the Critical Thinking Case Study (study guide, p. 33) ; then have them share their results with the class.

CLINICAL LABORATORY

1. With a client receiving an SSRI antidepressant drug, ask a student to interview the client regarding therapeutic and adverse effects. Results may be reviewed in a postconference discussion or written and turned in to the instructor.

2. For a client with a nursing diagnosis of Knowledge Deficit related to the effects and appropriate use of antidepressant drugs, have a student prepare a teaching plan.

3. Discuss ways to assist clients in maintaining usual activities of daily living (when feasible) while taking an antidepressant drug as an outpatient.

4. On a hospital unit with medical-surgical patients, assign one or more students to review medication administration records (MARs) and list the patients who are receiving an antidepressant. This exercise can increase students' awareness of depression as a common symptom among patients with nonpsychiatric illnesses.

5. In home care of a depressed client, have a student assess the risk of suicide, the ability and willingness to take antidepressant medication as prescribed, the use of other drugs that stimulate or depress CNS function, and the availability of social support systems. Have the student intervene (when indicated) to promote compliance, safety, and well-being.

■ Critical Thinking Case Study

1. A client admitted with depression is assessed for the following symptoms: loss of energy, fatigue, indecisiveness, difficulty thinking and concentrating, loss of interest in appearance, feelings of worthlessness, change in weight or appetite, sleep disorders, and obsession with death. The presence of 5 of these symptoms constitutes a major depression.

2. The 2 illnesses that should be considered before prescribing medication are diabetes mellitus and chronic lung disease. TCAs and lithium can cause weight gain, which could affect diabetic control. Continued smoking by an individual with chronic lung disease can decrease the effect of the TCAs. A diabetic taking MAO inhibitors can experience hypoglycemia. Persons with chronic lung disease can experience dyspnea as a result of SSRIs.

3. The client will experience improvement of mood. The client will resume self-care activities.

4. Teach clients to take antidepressant drugs as directed, that the therapeutic effects may not occur for 2–3 weeks, not to take other drugs without contacting their physician, and to tell other health care providers that they are taking this medication.

5. Observe for behaviors indicating lessening of depression, and observe for suicidal thoughts and behaviors. Also evaluate the client for weight loss.

6. Speak with the physician about the client's unwillingness and ask her the reason why she wants to discontinue the medication.

CHAPTER 11

Antiseizure Drugs

MAJOR TOPICS

- Seizure disorders, epilepsy
- Types of antiseizure drugs
- Treatment of seizure disorders

QUICK REFERENCE GUIDE TO TEXT

- Objectives, p. 169
- Interactive displays, pp. 169, 177, and 181
- Client teaching guidelines: Antiseizure medications, p. 178
- Table 11-1. Antiseizure drugs, p. 172
- Nursing process, pp. 176 and 181
- Principles of therapy, p. 177
- Review and application exercises, p. 185

TERMS AND CONCEPTS

Convulsion	Seizure
Epilepsy	Status epilepticus
Gingival hyperplasia	

DRUG LIST

- Carbamazepine (Tegretol)
- Fosphenytoin (Cerebyx)
- Gabapentin (Neurontin)
- Phenytoin (Dilantin)
- Topiramate (Topamax)
- Valproic acid (Depakene, Depakote)

■ Teaching Strategies

CLASSROOM

1. Lecture/discussion regarding selected seizure disorders and antiseizure drugs.

2. Discuss advantages and disadvantages of the various drugs in terms of efficacy and adverse effects.

3. Discuss the rationale for using a single drug when possible (monotherapy versus polytherapy).

4. Contrast dosage and intravenous administration of phenytoin and fosphenytoin.

5. Discuss the importance of teaching clients receiving long-term antiseizure therapy not to stop taking their medication abruptly or without their physician's consent and supervision.

6. Describe the nursing care needed by a client experiencing an acute tonic-clonic convulsion.

COLLABORATIVE ACTIVITIES FOR SMALL GROUPS

1. Assign groups to discuss review and application exercise number 3 (text, p. 185).

2. Ask groups to describe how they can identify clients who are at risk for status epilepticus and what interventions may be useful if status epilepticus occurs.

3. Assign groups to discuss the Critical Thinking Case Study (study guide, p. 38) and report their findings to the class.

CLINICAL LABORATORY

1. Ask students to identify clients who are at risk for acute seizures or status epilepticus.

2. For clients receiving an antiseizure drug, have students assess perceptions of the disease process, the prescribed drug therapy, and compliance with the prescribed treatment regimen.

3. For clients receiving an antiseizure drug, have students verbalize at least 1 nursing diagnosis related to drug therapy.

4. For clients known to have epilepsy, have students assess the ability of family members or caregivers to recognize and appropriately manage an acute seizure.

5. Determine the agency's procedure for rapidly obtaining intravenous diazepam or lorazepam when a patient has a convulsion or status epilepticus. In postconference discussions, review the procedure and have students role play the nursing process for a patient experiencing a tonic-clonic seizure.

6. If able to obtain a vial of phenytoin and a vial of fosphenytoin, have students read the labels of each medication and describe preparation and intravenous administration of a particular dose.

■ Critical Thinking Case Study

1. Stay with her and prevent her from hurting herself. Make sure that she can breathe adequately; time and observe the characteristics of the seizure.

2. The larger the anticonvulsant dose, the greater the possibility of adverse effects. Therefore, the physician has chosen to use 2 anticonvulsants at lower doses to control her seizures.

3. Contact her physician immediately. One or both of the medications may need to be discontinued.

4. There is no way of knowing at this time how long C.M. may need to be taking the medications. It is common practice to keep a patient on medication for 1 year after injury or until seizure free for 1 year. There is a possibility, depending on the extent of her injury, that C.M. may need to take the medication the rest of her life.

5. To reach a therapeutic serum level requires 2–3 weeks, and to achieve a steady-state concentration takes 3–4 weeks. Take the drug exactly as the doctor prescribes; it must not be stopped abruptly. Report any seizure activity or excessive drowsiness; the physician may need to adjust the drug dosage. Carry identification that contains the medical information that would be needed in the event a seizure took place in public or there was an emergency situation. See the dentist regularly. Take the medications with food to prevent gastrointestinal upsets.

CHAPTER 12

Antiparkinson Drugs

MAJOR TOPICS

- Parkinson's disease
- Types of antiparkinson drugs

QUICK REFERENCE GUIDE TO TEXT

- Objectives, p. 186
- Interactive displays, pp. 186, 189, and 190
- Table 12-1. Antiparkinson drugs, p. 188
- Nursing process, pp. 190 and 194
- Client teaching guidelines: Antiparkinson drugs, p. 191
- Principles of therapy, p. 192
- Review and application exercises, p. 197

TERMS AND CONCEPTS

Anticholinergic	Idiopathic
Bradykinesia	Spasticity
Dopaminergic	Tremors

DRUG LIST

- Levodopa/carbidopa (Sinemet)
- Pramipexole (Mirapex)
- Ropinirole (Requip)
- Selegiline (Eldepryl)
- Tolcapone (Tasmar)

■ Teaching Strategies

CLASSROOM

1. Describe the main characteristics of Parkinson's disease.

2. Discuss the dopaminergic and anticholinergic effects of antiparkinson drugs.

3. Contrast treatment of idiopathic and drug-induced parkinsonism.

COLLABORATIVE ACTIVITIES FOR SMALL GROUPS

1. Write names of selected drugs on small pieces of paper and have a student from each group extract a name. Then ask the group to list advantages and disadvantages of the drug.

2. Assign one third of the groups to discuss the client situation (text, p. 186), another third to discuss review and application exercises 4 and 5 (text, p. 197), and the final third to discuss the Critical Thinking Case Study (study guide, p. 41). Ask one or more groups in each subgroup to report their findings.

CLINICAL LABORATORY

1. For a client known to have Parkinson's disease, have a student assess for therapeutic and adverse effects of prescribed drugs.

2. For a client known to have Parkinson's disease, have a student assess for nonpharmacologic treatments (eg, physical therapy for gait training).

3. For a client receiving an older antipsychotic drug, have a student assess for signs and symptoms of parkinsonism.

■ Critical Thinking Case Study

1. Anticholinergic agents are commonly the drugs of choice when symptoms are relatively mild.

2. Adverse effects of the medication and nursing interventions:
   a. Tachycardia and palpitations usually are not serious; contact physician if problematic.
   b. For tremors and restlessness, contact physician to adjust dose.
   c. For sedation and drowsiness, if excessive, adjust dose.
   d. For constipation, treat with fluids, roughage, exercise, and laxatives.

3. Parkinson's disease progresses at different rates in different individuals. The symptoms can be controlled with medications.

4. Levodopa and carbidopa are the drugs of choice when bradykinesia and rigidity are the predominant symptoms.

5. Assess vital signs, peripheral perfusion, lung sounds, urinary output, and renal function. Instruct the client not to stop the medication abruptly.

6. The following side effects can occur: dizziness, lightheadedness, insomnia (avoid driving), nausea (take with meals), weight loss, low blood pressure (change position slowly); use caution in extreme temperature.

CHAPTER 13

Skeletal Muscle Relaxants

MAJOR TOPICS

- Musculoskeletal pain and spasm
- Multiple sclerosis

QUICK REFERENCE GUIDE TO TEXT

- Objectives, p. 199
- Interactive displays, pp. 199 and 202
- Nursing process, pp. 200 and 203
- Table 13-1. Skeletal muscle relaxants, p. 201
- Client teaching guidelines: Skeletal muscle relaxants, p. 202
- Principles of therapy, p. 202
- Review and application exercises, p. 204

TERMS AND CONCEPTS

Clonic	Spasticity
Malignant hyperthermia	Tonic
Muscle spasm	

DRUG LIST

- Baclofen (Lioresal)
- Carisoprodol (Rela, Soma)
- Dantrolene (Dantrium)
- Diazepam (Valium)

■ Teaching Strategies

CLASSROOM

1. Discuss acute musculoskeletal injury (eg, ankle sprain) and multiple sclerosis as conditions in which these drugs are used.

2. Discuss nonpharmacologic treatments of muscle spasm, musculoskeletal pain, and spasticity.

3. Differentiate between centrally active and peripherally active drugs.

4. Assign groups to discuss the Critical Thinking Case Study (study guide, p. 45).

CLINICAL LABORATORY

1. For a client with a nursing diagnosis of Self-Care Deficit related to spasm and pain, list the interventions needed.

2. For a client with multiple sclerosis, assess comfort level and functional ability in usual activities of daily living.

3. Interview a client with multiple sclerosis regarding his or her perceptions of "helping behaviors" from nurses and other health care providers.

■ Critical Thinking Case Study

1. Assess his mobility and pain level. Look for any swelling or tenderness. Ask him if he has been following the doctor's directions.

2. This medication is for short-term use. The maximum recommended duration is 3 weeks.

3. Other therapies include moist heat, massage, exercise, relaxation techniques, and NSAIDs.

CHAPTER 14

Anesthetics

MAJOR TOPICS

- Types of anesthesia
- General and local anesthetics
- Perioperative adjunctive drugs
- Nurse's role in preoperative and postoperative care

QUICK REFERENCE GUIDE TO TEXT

- Objectives, p. 205
- Interactive displays, pp. 205 and 212
- Table 14-1. General anesthetics, p. 208
- Table 14-2. Neuromuscular blocking agents, p. 210
- Table 14-3. Local anesthetics, p. 211
- Nursing process, pp. 212 and 217
- Client teaching guidelines: Perioperative medications, p. 213
- Client teaching guidelines: Topical anesthetics, p. 213
- Principles of therapy, p. 214
- Review and application exercises, p. 222

TERMS AND CONCEPTS

Adjunctive medications
Epidural anesthesia
General anesthesia

Postanesthesia recovery
Regional anesthesia

■ Teaching Strategies

CLASSROOM

1. Lecture/discussion of types and characteristics of general and regional anesthesia.

2. Ask students for personal experiences or their observations of clients before and after surgery.

3. Describe the appearance and care of a client in the immediate postoperative period after general inhalational anesthesia.

COLLABORATIVE ACTIVITIES FOR SMALL GROUPS

1. Assign groups to discuss the client care situation (text, p. 205).

2. Assign groups to discuss the Critical Thinking Case Study (study guide, p. 48).

CLINICAL LABORATORY

1. For a postoperative client, have a student review operative records, list preoperative medications, list anesthetic and other intraoperative drugs, and discuss implications for postoperative nursing care.

2. In an ambulatory surgery center or emergency room, have a student observe or assist with a minor procedure requiring local anesthesia.

■ Critical Thinking Case Study

1. Other situations in which this type of anesthesia may be used include perineal and rectal surgery.

2. What Mrs. J. will be able to feel depends on the sites of injection and the level to which the drug

rises in the spinal column. It will be a number of hours before Mrs. J. will have full mobility and sensation in her lower extremities.

3. The duration of the block can vary depending on the type of block and the drug concentration. When you feel an urge to void, call the nurse to assist you, because hypotension can occur after spinal anesthesia.

4. The fetal responses to anesthesia may include depressed muscle strength, muscle tone, and rooting behavior.

5. The infant should be assessed regularly after delivery. The depressed rooting behavior may make breastfeeding more challenging initially, and the mother should be reassured that this situation is temporary.

6. Urinary retention is common after spinal surgery. The nurse should assess Mrs. J. for bladder distention. If she has been NPO for a number of hours, she may not need to void at this time. If her bladder is distended and she is uncomfortable, contact the physician.

CHAPTER 15

Substance Abuse Disorders

MAJOR TOPICS

- Drug abuse and dependence
- Physiologic effects of alcohol, cocaine, marijuana, and nicotine
- Withdrawal reactions
- Treatment of abuse and dependence

QUICK REFERENCE GUIDE TO TEXT

- Objectives, p. 223
- Interactive displays, pp. 223 and 235
- Table 15-1. Drugs used to treat substance abuse disorders, p. 226
- Box 15-1. Effects of alcohol abuse, p. 227
- Box 15-2. Effects of cocaine abuse, p. 231
- Box 15-3. Effects of nicotine, p. 232
- Box 15-4. Effects of marijuana, p. 233
- Nursing process, p. 235
- Principles of therapy, p. 236
- Review and application exercises, p. 237

TERMS AND CONCEPTS

Alcohol abuse	Hallucinogen
Drug abuse	Physical dependence
Drug withdrawal reactions	Psychological dependence

DRUG LIST

- Cocaine
- Disulfiram (Antabuse)
- Ethanol
- Heroin
- Levo-alpha-acetylmethadol (LAAM) (Orlaam)
- Marijuana
- Naltrexone (ReVia)
- Nicotine (Nicoderm, Nicorette)

■ Teaching Strategies

CLASSROOM

1. Discuss assessment of clients in relation to risk for abuse of drugs.
2. Discuss management of clients with acute or chronic alcohol intoxication.
3. Discuss the rationale for administering sedatives to clients with alcohol dependence.
4. Review administration of flumazenil and naloxone.
5. Discuss nurses as a high-risk group for abuse of drugs.
6. Discuss ethical and legal implications of nurses who divert clients' drugs to themselves.
7. Discuss ethical and legal implications for nurses who suspect another nurse (a coworker) is abusing drugs.
8. Discuss the use of LAAM or methadone in the treatment of heroin addiction.
9. Discuss the use of nicotine replacement in smoking cessation regimens.

COLLABORATIVE ACTIVITIES FOR SMALL GROUPS

1. Have students discuss circumstances that might cause a nurse to take mind-altering drugs that have not been prescribed for him or her.

2. If a nurse suspects that a nursing colleague is taking a patient's opioid analgesic, does the patient or the colleague take priority in the nurse's consideration? Have students debate and justify their opinions about this situation.

3. Assign groups to discuss the client care situation (text, p. 223) or the Critical Thinking Case Study (study guide, p. 52).

CLINICAL LABORATORY

1. For a client who is receiving benzodiazepines or opiates, assign a student to assess for manifestations of abuse, dependence, and overdose.

2. For a client who acts intoxicated during hospitalization, review medical records and interview visitors to assess prehospitalization behavior and possible causes of the behavior.

3. In organized health care settings, review agency policies about the handling of psychotropic and narcotic drugs.

4. In home care settings, assess all members of the household in relation to possible abuse of alcohol or other drugs.

■ Critical Thinking Case Study

1. The nurse needs to identify health problems, allergies, medications, and social habits, including daily alcohol and drug intake. The nurse should also find out whether M. is being monitored by a physician.

2. Ingestion of alcohol during pregnancy can cause fetal alcohol syndrome.

3. M. is symptomatic and needs to be medicated. Normally benzodiazepines such as Librium are used to prevent delirium tremens. Any medication administered during pregnancy must be evaluated for its detrimental effects on the fetus.

4. Delirium tremens is characterized by confusion, disorientation, delusion, and hallucinations.

5. Antepartum care should be discussed, including proper nutrition. M.'s smoking habit also needs to be addressed because of its harmful effects on the fetus.

6. Referrals the nurse should make include the health department/visiting nurse association, an alcoholic rehabilitation program, and a physician for follow-up.

7. If alcohol is ingested concurrently with Antabuse, flushing, dyspnea, hypotension, tachycardia, nausea, vomiting, syncope, vertigo, blurred vision, headache, confusion, respiratory depression, dysrhythmia, myocardial infarction, unconsciousness, convulsions, or death can occur. The same type of reaction can also occur when certain drugs are ingested with Antabuse.

CHAPTER 16

Central Nervous System Stimulants

MAJOR TOPICS

- Amphetamines and related drugs
- Disorders for which CNS stimulants are used

QUICK REFERENCE GUIDE TO TEXT

- Objectives, p. 239
- Interactive displays, p. 239
- Nursing process, pp. 241 and 243
- Client teaching guidelines: Methylphenidate, p.242
- Principles of therapy, p. 242
- Review and application exercises, p. 244

TERMS AND CONCEPTS

Attention deficit-hyperactivity disorder (ADHD)
Narcolepsy

DRUG LIST

- Caffeine
- Dextroamphetamine (Dexedrine)
- Methylphenidate (Ritalin)

■ Teaching Strategies

CLASSROOM

1. Some authorities think ADHD is too frequently diagnosed and treated with CNS stimulants. Assign two groups of students to debate this issue.

2. Discuss potential therapeutic and adverse effects of CNS stimulant therapy in children.

3. Discuss ethical implications of using Ritalin in preschool children.

CLINICAL LABORATORY

1. In a school, outpatient clinic, or physician's office, observe a child diagnosed with ADHD and compare his or her behavior with the behavior of a similar-aged child without ADHD.

2. Prepare a teaching plan for the parents of a child for whom methylphenidate has been newly prescribed for ADHD.

DRUGS AFFECTING THE AUTONOMIC NERVOUS SYSTEM

CHAPTER 17

Physiology of the Autonomic Nervous System

MAJOR TOPICS

- General characteristics and functions of the sympathetic nervous system (SNS)
- General characteristics and functions of the parasympathetic nervous system (PNS)
- Overview of autonomic nervous system (ANS) drugs

QUICK REFERENCE GUIDE TO TEXT

- Objectives, p. 249
- Figure 17-1. Autonomic and somatic nervous systems, p. 250
- Figure 17-2. Signal transduction mechanism, p. 252
- Table 17-1. Adrenergic receptors, p. 253
- Review and application exercises, p. 255

TERMS AND CONCEPTS

Acetylcholine	Norepinephrine
Adrenergic	Parasympatholytic
Alpha-adrenergic receptors	Parasympathomimetic
Anticholinergic	Stress response
Beta-adrenergic receptors	Sympatholytic
Catecholamines	Sympathomimetic
Cholinergic	

■ Teaching Strategies

CLASSROOM

1. Student knowledge about the ANS, including receptors, is essential to understanding how drugs increase or decrease ANS functions. Therefore, a relatively detailed review and discussion may be needed.

2. Show a transparency of Figure 17-1 (text, p. 250; transparency 16) to review characteristics of the ANS.

3. Show a transparency of Figure 17-2 (text, p. 252; transparency 18) to illustrate cellular effects of beta-adrenergic receptor activation.

4. To focus students' attention, have them count their own heart rates while seated, stand and do "jumping jack" exercises for 2–3 minutes, then count their heart rates again. Ask "What have we done in relation to today's topic?" The answer is, "We've activated our sympathetic nervous systems." Discussion about effects of SNS stimulation can proceed.

5. Show a transparency of Table 17-1 (text, p. 253; transparency 17) to provide an overview of adrenergic receptors and the consequences of their activation.

CLINICAL LABORATORY

1. Ask students to assess assigned clients for signs and symptoms of SNS stimulation (stress response or "fight or flight" reaction).

2. Ask students to assess assigned clients for signs and symptoms of PNS stimulation.

CHAPTER **18**

Adrenergic Drugs

MAJOR TOPICS

- Adrenergic receptors
- Epinephrine as the prototype of adrenergic drugs
- Multipurpose adrenergic drugs

QUICK REFERENCE GUIDE TO TEXT

- Objectives, p. 256
- Interactive displays, pp. 256 and 261
- Table 18-1. Adrenergic drugs, p. 257
- Nursing process, pp. 261 and 265
- Client teaching guidelines: Adrenergic drugs, p. 262
- Principles of therapy, p. 263
- Review and application exercises, p. 269

TERMS AND CONCEPTS

Alpha-adrenergic receptors	Dopamine
Beta-adrenergic receptors	Norepinephrine
Bronchoconstriction	Vasoconstriction
Bronchospasm	Vasodilation

DRUG LIST

- Epinephrine (Adrenalin)
- Phenylephrine (Neo-Synephrine)
- Phenylpropanolamine (Propagest, Acutrim, others)
- Pseudoephedrine (Sudafed, others)

■ Teaching Strategies

CLASSROOM

1. Discuss common conditions for which adrenergic drugs are used.
2. Ask students about their experiences with conditions for which the drugs are used.

COLLABORATIVE ACTIVITIES FOR SMALL GROUPS

1. Assign groups to discuss uses of the drugs in various situations and populations (eg, management of toxicity and overdose in a child, young adult, or older adult; treatment of nasal congestion in a client with cardiovascular disease) (see Principles of Therapy, text, p. 263).
2. Ask groups to discuss review and application exercises 3, 5, and 7 (text, p. 269).
3. Assign the Critical Thinking Case Study (study guide, p. 60).

CLINICAL LABORATORY

1. Show students the emergency drug supply. Have students select or name the adrenergic drugs and describe their preparation and administration in specific emergency situations (eg, anaphylactic shock, cardiopulmonary resuscitation).
2. For clients receiving an adrenergic drug, have students assess for therapeutic and adverse effects.
3. For clients receiving an adrenergic drug, have students assess for conditions that may be aggravated by use of adrenergic drugs. If such conditions are found, assign students to teach the clients to avoid OTC appetite suppressants, asthma

remedies (bronchodilators), nasal decongestants, and multisymptom cold remedies containing decongestants.

▪ Critical Thinking Case Study

1. Epinephrine (Adrenalin) is a cardiac stimulant, vasopressor, and bronchodilator. Aminophylline is a bronchodilator. Corticosteroids decrease the inflammatory process.

2. Nursing assessments include vital signs and ECG findings, because epinephrine increases the heart rate. Anxiety and emotional changes can occur because of sympathetic nervous system stimulation. Assess urinary output, because epinephrine can constrict renal blood flow and decrease urine formation.

3. Antihistamines are used for allergic reactions that are not severe.

CHAPTER 19

Antiadrenergic Drugs

MAJOR TOPICS

- Differentiation of effects of alpha-adrenergic agonists and blocking agents
- Beta-adrenergic blocking agents
- Use of alpha- and beta-adrenergic blocking agents in cardiovascular and other disorders

QUICK REFERENCE GUIDE TO TEXT

- Objectives, p. 270
- Interactive displays, pp. 270, 277, and 278
- Figure 19-1. Action of beta-adrenergic blocking drugs, p. 271
- Table 19-1. Alpha-adrenergic agonists and blocking agents, p. 273
- Table 19-2. Beta-adrenergic blocking agents, p. 274
- Nursing process, pp. 277 and 281
- Client teaching guidelines: Alpha$_2$ agonists and alpha$_1$ blocking agents, p. 277
- Client teaching guidelines: Beta blocking agents, p. 278
- Principles of therapy, p. 278
- Review and application exercises, p. 284

TERMS AND CONCEPTS

Alpha agonists and blocking agents

Beta-adrenergic blocking agents

Benign prostatic hyperplasia

Cardioselective

DRUG LIST

- Atenolol (Tenormin)
- Clonidine (Catapres)
- Labetalol (Normodyne, Trandate)
- Metoprolol (Lopressor)
- Doxazosin (Cardura)
- Propranolol (Inderal)
- Terazosin (Hytrin)

■ Teaching Strategies

CLASSROOM

1. The concept that alpha$_2$-adrenergic agonists (eg, clonidine and related drugs) have antiadrenergic effects may be confusing. To aid student understanding of drug action, emphasize that the drugs cause less norepinephrine to be released at presynaptic nerve endings.

2. Lecture/discussion about the effects and uses of alpha$_1$-adrenergic blocking agents (transparency 19).

3. Discuss effects of beta blockers in relation to the disorders for which the drugs are used and in relation to adverse drug reactions.

4. Show transparencies of Figure 19-1 (text, p. 271; transparency 21) and of nonselective and cardioselective beta blockers (transparency 20). To aid recognition, remind students that generic names of beta blockers end in "-lol."

5. Show a transparency of the cardiovascular indications for use of beta blockers (transparency 22).

COLLABORATIVE ACTIVITIES FOR SMALL GROUPS

1. If not assigned as homework, have students complete the true-false exercise on beta blockers (study guide, p. 61). This can also be displayed as a transparency and completed by the group of students.

2. Assign groups to prepare a teaching plan for a client starting an alpha$_2$ agonist, an alpha$_1$ blocking agent, or a beta blocker.

3. Assign students to write answers to the review and application exercises (text, p. 284).

4. Assign the Critical Thinking Case Study (study guide, p. 64) for a few minutes, then discuss with entire class.

CLINICAL LABORATORY

1. For a client with a clonidine transdermal patch, ask a student to
   a. Consult a drug reference about application and effects (if new to the student).
   b. Interview the client about application and effects.
   c. Compare the client's statements with information in the drug reference and evaluate for discrepancies.
   d. Resolve any discrepancies found.
   e. Accurately apply the patch if indicated.
   f. Share information and administration techniques with the clinical group in preconference or postconference discussions.

2. For a client taking an alpha$_1$ blocker, have a student monitor blood pressure and assess for dizziness after drug administration.

3. For a client taking a beta blocker, have a student check heart rate and evaluate whether the value obtained is a therapeutic or adverse effect.

4. Ask students how they might reply when a client taking a beta blocker complains of fatigue.

5. Provide groups with a copy of agency instruction sheets related to alpha blockers and beta blockers and ask them to individualize instructions for particular clients.

CHAPTER 20

Cholinergic Drugs

MAJOR TOPICS

- Alzheimer's disease
- Clinical uses of cholinergic drugs
- Limitations of cholinergic drugs

QUICK REFERENCE GUIDE TO TEXT

- Objectives, p. 286
- Interactive displays, pp. 286 and 289
- Nursing process, pp. 289 and 292
- Client teaching guidelines: Cholinergic drugs, p. 290
- Principles of therapy, p. 290
- Review and application exercises, p. 294

TERMS AND CONCEPTS

Acetylcholine

Acetylcholinesterase

Cholinergic

Myasthenia gravis

Urinary retention

DRUG LIST

- Bethanechol (Urecholine)
- Donepezil (Aricept)
- Neostigmine (Prostigmin)

■ Teaching Strategies

CLASSROOM

1. Because these drugs are rarely used in most settings, the instructor may choose to assign portions of the chapter to be studied independently, to emphasize a few main points in lecture, or to prepare a written handout that summarizes drug effects.

2. Discuss the prevalence of Alzheimer's disease, the limitations of current drug therapy, and the need for effective drugs.

CLINICAL LABORATORY

1. For a client who has had thoracic or abdominal surgery, ask a student to check the operative record for administration of a cholinergic agent used to reverse effects of a neuromuscular blocking agent.

2. For a client with myasthenia gravis, ask a student to list the cholinergic drug, evaluate the dose in relation to literature recommendations, and interview the client about signs and symptoms of too much or too little drug.

3. For a client with Alzheimer's disease who is receiving donepezil, assess the client or interview caregivers about therapeutic and adverse drug effects.

■ Critical Thinking Case Study

1. J. has undergone abdominal surgery, during which he received general anesthesia, which decreases bowel function. His bowel was also manipulated

during the procedure. His bowel sounds should return in 24–48 hours. Activity usually enhances the return of bowel sounds.

2. J.'s NG tube is suctioning hydrochloric acid out of his stomach, which can cause alkalosis and hypokalemia.

3. The physician ordered Urecholine to increase tone and contractility of gastrointestinal and bladder smooth muscle. The recommended pediatric dose is 0.1 mg/kg and may be increased up to 0.4 mg/kg every 4 hours. J. weighs 30 kg. Therefore the recommended dose would be 3 mg.

4. J. should have decreased abdominal distention, have audible bowel sounds, and be able to void adequate amounts of urine without difficulty.

5. Hypotension, miosis, and increased perspiration are adverse effects of cholinergic drugs. The nurse should also assess J. for symptoms of infection, because J. is tachycardic and his temperature is elevated. The next dose of Urecholine should be held, and his physician should be contacted.

6. A cholinergic crisis can precipitate respiratory failure. Atropine is the antidote for cholinergic agents.

CHAPTER 21

Anticholinergic Drugs

MAJOR TOPICS

- Effects of anticholinergic drugs on body tissues
- Indications and limitations on clinical use of anticholinergic drugs
- Use of atropine as an antidote for cholinergic poisoning
- Management of anticholinergic overdose

QUICK REFERENCE GUIDE TO TEXT

- Objectives, p. 295
- Interactive displays, pp. 295 and 301
- Table 21-1. Tertiary and quaternary amine drugs, p. 296
- Nursing process, pp. 299 and 303
- Client teaching guidelines: Anticholinergic drugs, p. 300
- Principles of therapy, p. 301
- Review and application exercises, p. 305

TERMS AND CONCEPTS

Antispasmodic	Mydriasis
Cycloplegia	Parasympatholytic
Heat stroke	Vagal stimulation

DRUG LIST

- Atropine sulfate
- Glycopyrrolate (Robinul)

■ Teaching Strategies

CLASSROOM

1. Review selected effects of acetylcholine.
2. Explain that the effects of anticholinergic drugs stem directly from their ability to block acetylcholine receptors in various body tissues.
3. Discuss the Critical Thinking Case Study (study guide, p. 70).

CLINICAL LABORATORY

1. For clients receiving one or more drugs with anticholinergic effects, have students assess for therapeutic and adverse drug effects.
2. Discuss nursing interventions that prevent or decrease dry mouth, urinary retention, and tachycardia associated with systemic anticholinergic drugs.

■ Critical Thinking Case Study

1. The confusion could be a reaction to the atropine. The nurse should perform a complete assessment, including assessing vital signs, laboratory values (creatinine, digoxin level, electrolytes, hemoglobin), O_2 saturation, and neurologic checks, to help determine the cause of the confusion. The physician should be made aware of the change in the client's status.
2. The dry mouth and blurred vision are related to administration of atropine and will subside.
3. A pacemaker treats electrical conduction failure and causes the heart to beat at a regular rate, but it does not cure heart failure. Mr. P. will probably continue to take medications for his heart failure.

DRUGS AFFECTING THE ENDOCRINE SYSTEM

CHAPTER 22

Physiology of the Endocrine System

MAJOR TOPICS

- Endocrine-nervous system interactions
- Hormone pharmacokinetics
- Hormone actions at the cellular level
- Hormonal disorders
- General characteristics of hormonal drugs

QUICK REFERENCE GUIDE TO TEXT

- Objectives, p. 309
- Box 22-1. Major hormones, p. 310
- Review and application exercises, p. 313

TERMS AND CONCEPTS

Hormone
Hypothalamic-pituitary-adrenocortical (HPA) axis
Negative feedback system
Second messenger systems

■ Teaching Strategies

CLASSROOM

1. Ask students to define "hormone" and ask additional questions to determine what students already know about hormones.
2. Discuss review and application exercises 2 and 4 (text, p. 313).

CLINICAL LABORATORY

1. Have students identify and assess assigned clients for hormone imbalance.
2. For a client receiving a hormonal drug, ask students to determine whether the dose is physiologic or pharmacologic.

CHAPTER 23

Hypothalamic and Pituitary Hormones

MAJOR TOPICS

- Hypothalamus and its secretions
- Pituitary gland and its secretions

QUICK REFERENCE GUIDE TO TEXT

- Objectives, p. 314
- Interactive displays, pp. 314 and 319
- Nursing process, pp. 318 and 319
- Principles of therapy, p. 319
- Review and application exercises, p. 322

TERMS AND CONCEPTS

Adrenocorticotropic
  hormone (ACTH)
Antidiuretic hormone
  (ADH)
Corticotropin
Gonadotropin
Growth hormone

Oxytocin
Releasing hormone
Somatotropin
Thyroid-stimulating
  hormone
Thyrotropin

DRUG LIST

- Growth hormone (somatrem, somatropin)
- Oxytocin (Pitocin)

■ Teaching Strategies

CLASSROOM

1. Discuss reasons for the infrequent use of hypothalamic and pituitary hormones in clinical practice.

2. Discuss growth hormone as an example of a hormone affecting essentially all body cells.

3. Describe characteristics of a young child that may indicate inadequate endogenous growth hormone.

CLINICAL LABORATORY

1. In a medical-surgical setting, discuss the advantages of administering an adrenal corticosteroid rather than corticotropin (ACTH).

2. In an obstetric setting, review the dose, route, and specific monitoring of a client receiving oxytocin to induce or augment the labor process.

■ Critical Thinking Case Study

1. This medication will increase the force of your contractions and help your labor progress.

2. There must be continuous monitoring of uterine contractions, fetal and maternal heart rates, and maternal blood pressure and respiratory rate. The physician should be notified if contractions last longer than 1 minute or occur more frequently than every 2 minutes. Intake and output should also be monitored.

3. The Pitocin is increased slowly to allow for a gradual increase in uterine contractions.

4. Encourage Ms. G. to use the relaxation techniques she learned during prenatal classes. Contact her physician to see whether he will allow her to have pain medications.

5. Pitocin is continued after delivery for many individuals to control uterine bleeding.

CHAPTER 24

Corticosteroids

MAJOR TOPICS

- Endogenous corticosteroids: secretion and effects
- Differentiation of glucocorticoid and mineralocorticoid effects
- Exogenous corticosteroids; use in various conditions
- Preventing adrenal crisis

QUICK REFERENCE GUIDE TO TEXT

- Objectives, p. 323
- Interactive displays, pp. 323, 332, and 340
- Box 24-1. Effects of glucocorticoids, p. 325
- Box 24-2. Effects of mineralocorticoids, p. 326
- Table 24-1. Corticosteroid drugs, p. 329
- Nursing process, pp. 332 and 341
- Client teaching guidelines: Long-term corticosteroids, p. 334
- Principles of therapy, p. 336
- Review and application exercises, p. 344

TERMS AND CONCEPTS

Addison's disease	Glucocorticoid
Adrenocortical insufficiency	Immunosuppressive
Cushing's disease	Mineralocorticoid

DRUG LIST

- Beclomethasone (Beclovent, Vanceril, Vancenase)
- Dexamethasone (Decadron)
- Fluticasone (Flonase)
- Hydrocortisone
- Methylprednisolone (Medrol, others)
- Prednisone

■ Teaching Strategies

CLASSROOM

1. Because of the importance and frequent clinical use of these drugs, this content may warrant a couple of class periods.

2. The objectives may be used as an outline for lecture/discussion. Discuss hydrocortisone as the prototypical drug and the others as commonly used drugs in a variety of clinical settings.

3. Emphasize that many corticosteroids are available in several different formulations, for various indications and routes of administration. These formulations are not interchangeable and should be used solely for their designated purpose or route.

4. Ask students to share their previous experiences with clients receiving corticosteroids.

COLLABORATIVE ACTIVITIES FOR SMALL GROUPS

1. Have students prepare a teaching plan for long-term prednisone therapy, using the client teaching guidelines (text, p. 335) and a pharmacy instruction sheet for prednisone, from a hospital or community pharmacy.

2. Choose various formulations, routes of administration, conditions, and populations (see Principles of Therapy, text, p. 336). Then, assign groups to discuss, list the main points related to corticosteroid use, and share their findings with the class as a whole. This exercise could help students

see, for example, the differences in drug use between acute and chronic asthma and the differences between local and systemic effects.

3. Have students discuss one or more of review questions 6 through 10, and randomly select groups to report their findings to the entire class.

4. Assign the client situation (text, p. 323) for discussion. Ask groups to write or verbally report their opinions, with rationale.

5. Assign the Critical Thinking Case Study (study guide, p. 81) as homework to be turned in. This will assist in evaluating student understanding of corticosteroid therapy.

CLINICAL LABORATORY

1. Have students administer corticosteroids by oral, intravenous, inhalation, and topical routes when opportunities arise. In clinical conferences, discuss advantages and disadvantages of various routes.

2. For clients receiving a corticosteroid drug, discuss the reason for use, the route of administration, and the expected effects in each client.

3. For clients receiving long-term corticosteroid therapy, have students assess for edema, increased blood pressure, bruised skin, hypokalemia, hyperglycemia, and other adverse effects.

4. Review agency instruction sheets for various corticosteroids and ask students to individualize them for assigned clients.

■ Critical Thinking Case Study

1. G.'s mother should be aware of G.'s nutritional needs. She may need to increase the K^+ and Ca^{++} in his diet. G. will have an increased appetite, so she will need to provide low-calorie snacks to prevent excessive weight gain. Corticosteroid use can cause growth retardation, and G.'s mother needs to know this. Hyperglycemia is an adverse effect of the medication, so his blood sugar will need to be monitored routinely. G. will also be more susceptible to infection, so G.'s mother needs to monitor any cuts or abrasions and observe for any symptoms of infection.

2. At this point there is no way of knowing how long the treatment will be. Tests will be performed at various times over several weeks. Her son will be monitored very closely.

3. It would probably be helpful for her son to talk to a counselor about his feelings. It may be helpful to talk to the guidance counselor and teacher and have them speak to the children. It may also be helpful for him to talk to another child who has the same condition. Encourage G.'s mother to ask the physician for information regarding the length of treatment. G. may also need to be on a stricter diet with daily exercise.

CHAPTER 25

Thyroid and Antithyroid Drugs

MAJOR TOPICS

- Effects of thyroid disorders on body systems
- Hyperthyroidism
- Hypothyroidism
- Effects of thyroid disorders on metabolism of drugs

QUICK REFERENCE GUIDE TO TEXT

- Objectives, p. 346
- Interactive displays, pp. 346, 351, and 353
- Table 25-1. Effects of thyroid disorders, p. 348
- Client teaching guidelines: Thyroxine, p. 352
- Client teaching guidelines: Propylthiouracil, p. 353
- Nursing process, pp. 351 and 355
- Principles of therapy, p. 353
- Review and application exercises, p. 358

TERMS AND CONCEPTS

Cretinism   Thyroiditis
Graves' disease   Thyrotoxicosis
Myxedema   Thyroxine

DRUG LIST

- Levothyroxine (Synthroid)
- Propylthiouracil (Propacil)

◾ Teaching Strategies

CLASSROOM

1. Review the role of thyroid hormone in body metabolism.

2. Use Table 25-1 (text, p. 348) to demonstrate the generally opposing effects of hypothyroidism and hyperthyroidism.

3. Emphasize that drug therapy for 1 disorder may cause the other disorder.

COLLABORATIVE ACTIVITIES FOR SMALL GROUPS

1. Have students discuss the client scenario (text, p. 346) and prepare a teaching plan for the described client.

2. Assign selected review and application exercises (text, p. 358) for group discussion.

CLINICAL LABORATORY

1. For a client receiving levothyroxine or propylthiouracil, have a student assess for signs and symptoms of the disorder being treated (to evaluate therapeutic affects) and of the opposing disorder (to evaluate adverse effects).

2. Review laboratory reports of assigned clients for thyroid function tests (eg, TSH, T_3, T_4).

◾ Critical Thinking Case Study

1. The symptoms attributable to hyperthyroidism include weight loss, tachycardia, insomnia, and excessive perspiration.

2. Propylthiouracil is used to treat hyperthyroidism. Its therapeutic effect may not occur for days or weeks because of stored hormones. She will take the medication until her hyperthyroidism has been effectively treated. Propranolol (Inderal) is used for Mrs. G.'s tachycardia. She can begin to see therapeutic effects within 24–48 hours. It will be used to control tachycardia until the hyperthyroid symptoms are controlled.

3. When you are taking propylthiouracil (Propacil), you should observe for hypothyroidism, blood disorders, skin rashes, headache, dizziness, drowsiness, nausea, vomiting, abdominal discomfort, edema, joint pain, and drug fever. Inderal can cause hypotension, bronchospasm, dizziness, fatigue, depression, insomnia, and hallucinations. Since Mrs. G. was already having problems with insomnia, she should contact her physician if her insomnia does not get better or gets worse.

4. Hypothyroidism must be treated because it decreases all the functions of the body. The cardiovascular effects include decreased cardiac output, decreased heart rate, and heart failure.

5. Instruct Mrs. G. to take the medication as directed and not to discontinue it without consulting her physician. She should be instructed on how to check her pulse, and she should notify her physician if her resting pulse stays higher than 100 bpm or drops to less than 60 bpm. Advise her to notify her physician if headache, nervousness, diarrhea, excessive sweating, heat intolerance, chest pain, increased pulse rate, palpitations, weight loss (more than 2 lb/wk), or any unusual symptoms occur. Caution her to avoid taking other medications unless instructed by her physician. Instruct her to inform any other physicians or dentists of her thyroid therapy. Emphasize the importance of follow-up examinations.

CHAPTER 26

Hormones That Regulate Calcium and Bone Metabolism

MAJOR TOPICS

- Parathyroid hormone, calcitonin, and vitamin D
- Calcium and phosphorus
- Hypocalcemia
- Hypercalcemia
- Osteoporosis

QUICK REFERENCE GUIDE TO TEXT

TERMS AND CONCEPTS

Bisphosphonates
Calciferol

Calcitonin
Tetany

DRUG LIST

- Alendronate (Fosamax)
- Calcitonin—human (Cibacalcin)
- Calcium carbonate (Os-Cal, Tums)
- Calcium chloride
- Calcitriol (Rocaltrol)

■ Teaching Strategies

CLASSROOM

1. Use the objectives as a guide for lecture/discussion. Show transparencies 23 and 24.

2. Ask students about their personal intake of calcium (eg, use of dairy products) and to evaluate their personal intake in relation to the recommended dietary intake.

3. Discuss reasons why adolescent and young adult women are considered to be at high risk for inadequate dietary intake of calcium.

4. Discuss ways for members of high-risk groups to increase their intake of calcium.

5. Describe the risk factors and potential consequences of osteoporosis.

COLLABORATIVE ACTIVITIES FOR SMALL GROUPS

1. Assign the client scenario related to osteoporosis (text, p. 359) and have students write responses to the 5 statements.

2. Assign review and application exercises 3 through 7 (text, p. 376).

CLINICAL LABORATORY

1. Have students assess clients in relation to their risks of developing hypocalcemia, hypercalcemia, or osteoporosis.

2. Have students list serum calcium levels from their patients' medical records and evaluate these in terms of implications for nursing care.

3. Review emergency drugs located in the clinical setting and determine which may be used in treating hypocalcemia or hypercalcemia.

4. For a patient receiving chemotherapy for cancer, review serum calcium reports and evaluate the patient's risks of developing hypercalcemia.

5. For a client with osteoporosis, develop a teaching plan to prevent falls and fractures.

■ Critical Thinking Case Study

1. The nurse will assess for problems associated with renal failure. The assessments include vital signs, urinary output, and weights. The nurse will also observe for symptoms of hyperkalemia and hypercalcemia, which include abdominal cramping, muscle weakness, ECG changes, lethargy, personality changes, confusion, and paresthesia.

2. Intravenous normal saline will increase the urinary calcium excretion. Concurrent administration of Lasix decreases the risk of fluid overload and enhances urinary excretion of calcium and potassium. Administration of prednisone also increases calcium and potassium loss.

3. A complete assessment will be done, including vital signs, breath sounds, and a neurologic examination. After completing the physical examination, you will read the nursing notes from dialysis and look at the laboratory findings. A big concern after dialysis is disequilibrium syndrome; if symptoms worsen, contact the dialysis nurse or physician.

4. Lasix should be administered as early in the day as possible to prevent nocturia. Electrolyte levels need to be monitored on a regular basis. Weekly weights should be taken to evaluate the effectiveness of the medication.

CHAPTER 27

Antidiabetic Drugs

MAJOR TOPICS

- Types of diabetes mellitus
- Complications of diabetes
- Metabolic effects of endogenous insulin
- Types and characteristics of exogenous insulin
- Types and characteristics of oral antidiabetic drugs

QUICK REFERENCE GUIDE TO TEXT

TERMS AND CONCEPTS

Diabetogenic
Glucagon
Hyperglycemia
Hypoglycemia
Insulin resistance
Lactic acidosis

Ketoacidosis
Neuropathy
Polydipsia
Polyphagia
Polyuria

DRUG LIST

- Regular and NPH insulins
- Insulin lispro (Humalog)
- Acarbose (Precose)
- Glipizide (Glucotrol)
- Glyburide (DiaBeta, Micronase)
- Metformin (Glucophage)
- Miglitol (Glyset)
- Pioglitazone (Actos)
- Repaglinide (Prandin)
- Rosiglitazone (Avandia)

■ Teaching Strategies

CLASSROOM

1. This content warrants one or more class periods, unless drug treatment of diabetes is extensively discussed in another nursing course. The objectives can be used as an outline for lecture/discussion.

2. Show a transparency of Figure 27-1 (text, p. 378; transparency 25) to aid understanding of insulin action and glucose metabolism.

3. Discuss regular insulin as the prototype and other insulins as modifications of regular insulin.

4. Discuss advantages and disadvantages of intensive insulin therapy.

5. Differentiate oral antidiabetic agents. Show a transparency of Figure 27-2 (text, p. 385; transparency 26).

6. Discuss the use of combinations of insulin and oral agents or two types of oral agents in treatment of type 2 diabetes.

7. Ask students to write out answers to the review and application exercises (text, p. 406) and turn them in. Grades, points, or credits are recommended because of the number of questions and the time and effort required.

8. Ask students about their experiences with family members or clients who have diabetes.

9. Ask a nurse-diabetes educator to speak to the class about assisting clients with their antidiabetic drugs and other aspects of managing diabetes.

10. Obtain patient-oriented pamphlets and newsletters from a local chapter of the American Diabetes Association and circulate them among class members to demonstrate a community resource.

11. Discuss teaching needs in relation to diet, exercise, and antidiabetic drugs; emphasize the need to include family members or significant others in teaching sessions.

COLLABORATIVE ACTIVITIES FOR SMALL GROUPS

1. Assign groups to discuss the client scenario (text, p. 377) and write responses to the 5 statements. (In class discussion after small group work, the instructor might ask students how their answers would differ if Ellen had type 2 diabetes instead of type 1).

2. Assign groups to prepare a teaching plan for a client taking NPH and regular insulin twice daily, a client taking a single oral drug (eg, a sulfonylurea), or a client taking a sulfonylurea with an alpha-glucosidase inhibitor or glitazone.

3. Divide review questions (text, p. 406) among several groups and have them write responses to be discussed with the entire class.

4. Assign groups to review and list the main elements of treatment for hypoglycemia and diabetic ketoacidosis.

5. Assign groups to discuss the use of insulin and oral antidiabetic drugs for clients with renal or hepatic impairment or critical illness.

CLINICAL LABORATORY

1. Have students measure blood glucose levels from themselves, other students, or clients.

2. Have students participate in teaching newly diagnosed diabetic clients and their families. Locate and discuss client-teaching materials available in a health care setting. If available, show patient education videotapes related to the disease process, nonpharmacologic treatment measures, and pharmacologic treatments.

3. Have students administer insulin.

4. Have students monitor clients' laboratory reports for glycosylated hemoglobin levels, when available, and discuss nursing process implications of normal and abnormal values.

5. For clients receiving 1 or more antidiabetic drugs, ask students to assess for risk and for signs and symptoms of hypoglycemia.

6. Have a dietitian speak to a clinical group about dietary counseling with a diabetic client and family members.

■ Critical Thinking Case Study

1. Mrs. J. needs to avoid concentrated sweets and should eat 4 to 6 small, balanced meals to maintain an adequate blood sugar level. Symptoms of hypoglycemia and hyperglycemia should be reviewed. She should also be taught how to handle her diabetes when she becomes ill.

2. Mrs. J. should be checking her blood glucose levels regularly, recording them, and sharing them with her physician so that her insulin dosage can be adjusted. Mrs. J. is experiencing hypoglycemia during the night; therefore, her evening dose of NPH may need to be decreased. She may also need to increase her caloric intake at night. You should also find out whether Mrs. J. is exercising in the evening.

3. Ask if he can get Mrs. J. to drink. If she can, he should use a high-carbohydrate drink. If she cannot drink and there is glucagon in the house, he should administer it. If neither of these is possible, he should immediately bring Mrs. J. to the emergency room.

4. The NPH level peaks in approximately 8 hours. If Mrs. P. is taking NPH insulin at suppertime (6 PM), it should peak at about 2 AM. Changing the NPH dose to 10 PM would make it peak at 6 AM.

CHAPTER 28

Estrogens, Progestins, and Oral Contraceptives

MAJOR TOPICS

- Functions of endogenous estrogens
- Drug formulations of estrogens and progestins

QUICK REFERENCE GUIDE TO TEXT

- Objectives, p. 407
- Interactive displays, pp. 407 and 416
- Box 28-1. Effects of endogenous estrogens, p. 409
- Table 28-1. Estrogen drugs, p. 411
- Table 28-2. Progestin drugs, p. 412
- Nursing process, pp. 412 and 418
- Table 28-3. Contraceptive drugs, p. 413
- Principles of therapy, p. 414
- Client teaching guidelines: Oral contraceptives, p. 415
- Client teaching guidelines: Estrogen replacement therapy, p. 415
- Review and application exercises, p. 420

TERMS AND CONCEPTS

Contraception	Menstrual disorders
Menopause	Ovulation
Menstrual cycle	Thromboembolic disorders

DRUG LIST

- Estrogens (Premarin, Estrace, Estraderm)
- Medroxyprogesterone (Provera)

■ Teaching Strategies

CLASSROOM

1. If oral contraceptives are included in a maternal-child nursing course, the instructor may wish to omit or minimize discussion in the pharmacology class.

2. Assign 2 groups of students to debate the issue of hormone replacement therapy (HRT) for menopausal women.

3. Discuss advantages and disadvantages of HRT.

COLLABORATIVE ACTIVITIES FOR SMALL GROUPS

1. Prepare a teaching plan for a perimenopausal woman starting on HRT.

2. Discuss the Critical Thinking Case Study (study guide, p. 95) related to oral contraceptives.

CLINICAL LABORATORY

1. For clients receiving estrogen or progesterone, have students assess age, reason for use, and current or potential adverse effects.

2. For clients receiving an oral contraceptive, have students assess for risk factors and for signs and symptoms of deep vein thrombosis.

3. For a 40-year-old woman with a recent hysterectomy and bilateral oophorectomy (surgical menopause), discuss teaching needs in relation to estrogen replacement therapy.

■ Critical Thinking Case Study

1. Factors that preclude the use of birth control pills include pregnancy, thromboembolic disorders (increase hepatic production of clotting factors), cancer (can stimulate tumor growth), hypertension (increases angiotensin and sodium and water retention), smoking in women older than 35 years of age (smoking causes increased platelet aggregation).

2. Before drug therapy is started, the client needs a comprehensive physical examination, including measurements of blood pressure and cholesterol and triglyceride levels.

3. Persons can experience weight gain and acne from taking oral contraceptives. Mrs. G. needs to continue to take the medication and should make an appointment with her physician. The physician may change her medication, which could alleviate the problem.

CHAPTER 29

Androgens and Anabolic Steroids

MAJOR TOPICS

- Functions of androgens
- Abuse of anabolic steroids

QUICK REFERENCE GUIDE TO TEXT

- Objectives, p. 422
- Interactive display, p. 422
- Box 29-1. Effects of testosterone, p. 424
- Table 29-1. Androgens, p. 425
- Nursing process, pp. 425 and 427
- Client teaching guidelines: Androgens, p. 426
- Principles of therapy, p. 426
- Review and application exercises, p. 428

TERMS AND CONCEPTS

Anabolism	Jaundice
Epiphyseal closure	Steroid hormone
Hirsutism	

DRUG LIST

- Danazol (Danocrine)
- Testosterone

■ Teaching Strategies

CLASSROOM

1. Because these drugs are rarely given in most clinical settings, the instructor may choose to omit them or minimize class time.

2. Review (or have students review independently) the physiologic effects of endogenous androgens.

3. Discuss the effects of androgens on women and children.

4. Ask students whether they know other students who take anabolic steroids. If so, ask them to share their observations about appearances and behaviors of the drug-takers and their thoughts about adverse effects of the drugs.

COLLABORATIVE ACTIVITIES FOR SMALL GROUPS

1. Discuss the client scenario (text, p. 422) related to anabolic steroid abuse.

2. Discuss review and application exercise number 5 (text, p. 428).

3. Discuss the Critical Thinking Case Study (study guide, p. 98).

CLINICAL LABORATORY

1. For women receiving danazol, have students assess for masculinizing effects.

2. For children receiving testosterone, ask students to assess the parents' knowledge about and willingness to comply with the recommendation for x-rays every 6 months.

■ Critical Thinking Case Study

1. As teenagers, you believe that there are benefits to steroid use. Yes, you can get some increase in muscle mass, strength, and weight. You also need

to be aware of the negative effects of steroid use, which far outweigh the positive effects. Large doses of steroids cause a variety of liver disorders that can lead to hemorrhage or liver failure. Behavioral changes have been documented, including aggressiveness, hostility, and combativeness. Dependence can occur, which is characterized by preoccupation with drug use, inability to stop taking the drugs, and withdrawal symptoms. Large doses of steroids can result in testicular atrophy, low sperm counts, and impotence in men, and there is an increased risk of cardiovascular disease. Severe acne can also occur.

2. Physical changes indicative of steroid use that the nurse could be assessing for include
   a. Deepened voice.
   b. Increased muscle mass (the nurse could measure muscle mass).
   c. Weight gain (the nurse could check students' weights and also vital signs for a possible increase in blood pressure due to fluid retention).
   d. Increased serum cholesterol levels (the nurse could monitor serum cholesterol levels).

NUTRIENTS, FLUIDS, AND ELECTROLYTES

CHAPTER 30

Nutritional Support Products and Drugs for Obesity

MAJOR TOPICS

- Nutrient needs
- Disorders of water, carbohydrates, proteins, and fats
- Fluid disorders
- Enteral and parenteral nutrition in special populations
- Overnutrition (obesity)
- Undernutrition

QUICK REFERENCE GUIDE TO TEXT

- Objectives, p. 431
- Interactive displays, pp. 431, 436, and 442
- Table 30-1. Water imbalances, p. 432
- Table 30-2. Carbohydrate, protein, and fat imbalances, p. 432
- Table 30-3. Types of intravenous fluids, p. 433
- Table 30-4. Enteral products for children, p. 434
- Table 30-5. Enteral products for adults, p. 435
- Table 30-6. Drugs for obesity, p. 437
- Nursing process, pp. 438 and 446
- Client/caregiver teaching guidelines: Nutritional supplements and tube feedings, p. 439
- Client teaching guidelines: Drugs that aid weight loss, p. 440

- Principles of therapy, p. 440
- Review and application exercises, p. 449

TERMS AND CONCEPTS

Anorexiants	Malabsorption
Body mass index	Obesity
Enteral nutrition	Parenteral nutrition

PRODUCT AND DRUG LIST

- Ensure
- Orlistat (Xenical)
- Osmolite
- Pancrelipase (Viokase)
- Phenylpropanolamine (Acutrim, Dexatrim)
- Pulmocare
- Sibutramine (Meridia)
- TraumaCal

■ Teaching Strategies

CLASSROOM

1. Differentiate between nursing and dietary responsibilities in nutritional assessment and teaching.

2. Ask students to compare enteral and parenteral nutrition in terms of convenience to the client, efficacy, and adverse effects.

3. Discuss nutritional support of clients with cancer.

4. Ask students how they feel about society's obsession with "thinness" and their reaction to obese people.

5. Ask students about their perceptions of effective and rational weight loss techniques.

COLLABORATIVE ACTIVITIES FOR SMALL GROUPS

1. Ask students to list all the ways they can think of (in 5 or 10 minutes) to decrease caloric intake and increase exercise. (In class discussion after the small group activity, the instructor might want to ask whether any of the identified techniques are unhealthy or irrational.)

2. Discuss review and application exercise number 9 (text, p. 450).

3. Discuss the Critical Thinking Case Study (study guide, p. 102).

CLINICAL LABORATORY

1. Have students assess all assigned clients for risks of fluid and nutritional imbalances.

2. Have the clinical group analyze weight and height (and/or calculate body mass index) of selected clients to assist in determining nutritional status.

3. Have the clinical group evaluate drugs ordered for a client in terms of potential interference with fluid and nutritional needs.

4. For a client receiving intravenous fluids, have students analyze the fluids and nutrients provided per 24 hours and compare them with recommended amounts.

5. For a client receiving central or peripheral parenteral nutrition, interview the client and demonstrate the apparatus to students. Discuss agency policies for site care.

6. For a client receiving a supplementary enteral feeding, have students analyze the amount taken in relation to the amount needed.

7. For a client receiving tube feedings, show students a container of the prescribed formula and ask them to analyze the feeding according to the types and amounts of nutrients provided per day. Ask them to evaluate the adequacy of formula and fluid intake.

■ Critical Thinking Case Study

1. Pulmocare was chosen because it is the supplemental feeding of choice for clients with chronic obstructive pulmonary disease (COPD). Because of the impaired breathing, these clients have difficulty eliminating sufficient quantities of CO_2, a waste product of carbohydrate metabolism. When CO_2 accumulates in the body, it can produce respiratory acidosis and eventually respiratory failure. Pulmocare contains more fat (55%) and less carbohydrates (28%) than most other formulas. Consequently, its metabolism produces less CO_2. It contains 1.5 cal/mL. Mr. J. is to receive 80 mL/hr of Pulmocare. Therefore, he will receive $80 \times 24 = 1920$ mL per 24 hr. His caloric intake will be: $1920 \times 1.5 = 2880$ cal/day. This 2880 cal/day is sufficient to maintain his present weight.

2. The nurse should be assessing for diarrhea, fluid volume deficit, hypernatremia, and aspiration of the formula into the lungs.

3. TPN is expensive, is irritating to the vessels, and can cause hyperglycemia and septicemia. It is useful for individuals who do not have a functioning gastrointestinal tract. Mr. J. was probably started on enteral feedings because they are inexpensive and convenient (a patient can easily be transferred home or to a long-term care facility).

4. Aspiration is a common problem associated with tube feedings. It can be prevented by proper positioning, checking for tube placement, checking residual stomach content, and giving feedings slowly. Dehydration is another problem. Unless otherwise indicated, all persons receiving tube feedings should receive 1500–2000 mL of water daily.

5. Diarrhea is usually attributed to the hypertonicity of the preparations. Diarrhea can be prevented by starting with small amounts of dilute solutions and gradually increasing to full strength. The nurse should assess Mr. J.'s skin and his laboratory values and notify the physician that Mr. J. is having diarrhea. The physician may decrease the strength of the tube feeding or order an antidiarrheal medication.

CHAPTER 31

Vitamins

MAJOR TOPICS

- Types, functions, requirements, and food sources of vitamins

QUICK REFERENCE GUIDE TO TEXT

- Objectives, p. 451
- Interactive displays, pp. 451, 459, and 462
- Table 31-1. Vitamins as nutrients, p. 452
- Nursing process, pp. 455 and 465
- Table 31-2. Vitamin imbalances, p. 456
- Table 31-3. Vitamin drug preparations, p. 459
- Client teaching guidelines: Vitamins, p. 461
- Principles of therapy, p. 461
- Review and application exercises, p. 467

TERMS AND CONCEPTS

Coenzyme	Megaloblastic anemia
Fat-soluble vitamins	Pernicious anemia
Megadose	Water-soluble vitamins

■ Teaching Strategies

CLASSROOM

1. Students who have had a nutrition class may need only to review basic content and some discussion of vitamins as drugs.
2. Discuss use of RDAs in personal life to promote health and well-being.
3. Review ways to cook and store food to retain vitamin content.

4. Discuss the pros and cons of taking vitamin supplements.

COLLABORATIVE ACTIVITIES FOR SMALL GROUPS

1. Have students analyze OTC multivitamin preparations (eg, adult and children's multivitamins and a prenatal vitamin) in relation to the RDAs for the intended population.
2. Discuss review and application exercise number 8 (text, p. 467).
3. Discuss the Critical Thinking Case Study (study guide, p. 105).

CLINICAL LABORATORY

1. Have students assess assigned clients for actual or potential vitamin deficiency.
2. Ask students to teach clients ways to increase their dietary intake of vitamins.
3. Encourage students to teach clients (and others) to avoid megadoses of any vitamins, whenever an opportunity arises.

■ Critical Thinking Case Study

1. This would include a complete assessment, as well as a complete blood panel, because all body systems can be affected by malnutrition.
2. Niacin is essential for glycolysis, fat synthesis, and fat metabolism; when niacin is lacking, the individual can develop pellagra. Thiamine is essential for energy production. A mild deficiency causes fatigue, anorexia, growth retardation,

depression, and irritability. A severe deficiency causes peripheral neuritis, personality disturbances, and heart failure. Folic acid is essential for metabolism, normal red blood cells, and growth. Megaloblastic anemia, impaired growth in children, and GI problems can result from a folic acid deficiency. Vitamins are administered parenterally if severe GI malabsorption exists or the disease is severe.

3. After discussing with Mr. B. the rationale for administering the medications, if he still refuses the injections, contact his physician. The medications can be given orally.

CHAPTER 32

Minerals and Electrolytes

MAJOR TOPICS

- Minerals as nutrients
- Deficiency and excess states of sodium, potassium, and magnesium
- Drugs used in treatment of deficiency and excess states
- Metal chelating agents

QUICK REFERENCE GUIDE TO TEXT

- Objectives, p. 468
- Interactive displays, pp. 468, 478, and 482
- Table 32-1. Minerals and electrolytes, p. 469
- Table 32-2. Sodium imbalances, p. 471
- Table 32-3. Potassium imbalances, p. 472
- Table 32-4. Magnesium imbalances, p. 473
- Table 32-5. Chloride imbalances, p. 473
- Table 32-6. Selected trace elements, p. 474
- Table 32-7. Iron imbalances, p. 477
- Nursing process, pp. 479 and 485
- Principles of therapy, p. 480
- Client teaching guidelines: Mineral supplements, p. 481
- Review and application exercises, p. 489

TERMS AND CONCEPTS

Acidosis	Hyperkalemia
Alkalosis	Hypokalemia
Chelating agents	Micronutrients
Electrolyte	

DRUG LIST

- Deferoxamine (Desferal)
- Ferrous sulfate ($FeSO_4$)
- Potassium chloride (KCl) (K-Dur, Klor-Con)
- Sodium polystyrene sulfonate (Kayexalate)
- Succinimide (Chemet)

■ Teaching Strategies

CLASSROOM

1. Compare potassium content in selected food sources, salt substitutes, and prescription KCl preparations.
2. Ask students about their experiences with clients who were receiving KCl.
3. Ask students about personal intake of iron and whether they think they receive an adequate amount.

COLLABORATIVE ACTIVITIES FOR SMALL GROUPS

1. Discuss and list main elements of review and application exercises 2 and 3 (text, p. 489).
2. Discuss and list main elements of review and application exercises 4, 5, and 6 (text, p. 489).

CLINICAL LABORATORY

1. Have students assess assigned clients in relation to electrolyte balance, including usual eating habits and laboratory reports of serum sodium, potassium, and magnesium.

2. For clients receiving a diuretic, have students check serum potassium before giving the drug.

3. Have students assess assigned clients for iron deficiency anemia, including serum iron and iron-binding capacity if available.

4. In a home care setting, assess the environment for risk factors related to overdoses of iron, lead, potassium, and other metals.

■ Critical Thinking Case Study

1. A client in renal failure requires a complete assessment because this disease affects every body system. Besides assessing orientation, vital signs, intake and output, weight, and presence of edema, the nurse must also monitor the client's cardiac status.

2. Dysrhythmias can occur with hyperkalemia, acidosis, alkalosis, and hypocalcemia. Because Mr. B. is being treated for acidosis, the nurse must monitor the electrolyte changes carefully. Sodium bicarbonate is used to treat acidosis but can produce alkalosis, and alkalosis causes hypocalcemia.

3. Your serum potassium levels are still very high. We must bring them down so that you will not have any heart problems. The medication that we are giving you acts in your colon, so if we give it rectally it will work more rapidly.

DRUGS USED TO TREAT INFECTIONS

CHAPTER 33

General Characteristics of Antimicrobial Drugs

MAJOR TOPICS

- Host defense mechanisms
- Common pathogenic microorganisms
- Antibiotic-resistant microorganisms
- Use of antimicrobial drugs in special populations

QUICK REFERENCE GUIDE TO TEXT

- Objectives, p. 493
- Box 33-1. Common bacterial pathogens, p. 495
- Box 33-2. Antibiotic-resistant staphylococci, streptococci, and enterococci, p. 499
- Figure 33-1. Actions of antibacterials on bacterial cells, p. 501
- Nursing process, pp. 502 and 503
- Client teaching guidelines: Antimicrobial drugs, p. 504
- Principles of therapy, p. 504
- Review and application exercises, p. 511

TERMS AND CONCEPTS

Aerobic	Drug resistance
Anaerobic	Narrow spectrum
Bactericidal	Nosocomial
Bacteriostatic	Phagocytosis
Broad spectrum	Prophylactic
Chemoprophylaxis	Pseudomembranous colitis
Culture and susceptibility studies	Superinfection

■ Teaching Strategies

CLASSROOM

1. Lecture/discussion using the objectives as an outline.

2. Discuss risk factors for developing an infection.

3. Discuss circumstances in which a person is likely to develop an infection with antibiotic-resistant microorganisms.

4. Show a transparency of Figure 33-1 (text, p. 501; transparency 27) to provide an overview of antibacterial drug actions.

5. Discuss the importance of taking antimicrobial drugs as prescribed and the potential consequences of *not* taking them as prescribed.

6. Discuss ways in which nurses can promote rational use of antimicrobial drugs.

7. Ask a pharmacist or infection control nurse to speak to the class about local patterns of microbial resistance to antibiotics, difficulties in treating infections caused by antibiotic-resistant microorganisms, and CDC or personal recommendations for preventing emergence of drug-resistant microorganisms.

8. Assign students to obtain, read, and write a summary of a journal article related to some aspect of preventing, recognizing, or managing infectious diseases. Ask that a copy of the article be submitted with the summary.

COLLABORATIVE ACTIVITIES FOR SMALL GROUPS

1. Assign 2 groups of students to debate the issue of antibiotic use (eg, "Resolved: Overuse and inappropriate use of antibiotics endangers the public health").

2. Assign groups to prepare a general teaching plan about an antibiotic.

3. Discuss and write answers to the review and application exercises (text, p. 511).

CLINICAL LABORATORY

1. For clients with increased risk of developing infection, have students plan and implement interventions to decrease the risk.

2. For clients with infections, ask students to verbalize assessment data, state at least 1 nursing diagnosis, and state interventions to protect themselves and others in the environment.

3. For clients receiving an antimicrobial drug, have students check culture and susceptibility reports (if available), look up the specific drug, and evaluate whether the ordered drug is appropriate for the particular client.

4. For clients receiving an antimicrobial drug, have students obtain a copy of an agency instruction sheet and individualize it for their clients.

5. Have students discuss the importance of taking antimicrobial drugs as prescribed.

6. In hospital settings with an infection control nurse, ask the nurse to conduct a postclinical conference about nurses' roles and responsibilities in infection control.

CHAPTER 34

Beta-Lactam Antibacterials: Penicillins, Cephalosporins, and Others

MAJOR TOPICS

- Characteristics of beta-lactam antibacterial drugs
- Evolution of subgroups of penicillins
- Beta-lactamase inhibitor drugs
- Comparison of penicillins and cephalosporins
- Similarities and differences between "generations" of cephalosporins

QUICK REFERENCE GUIDE TO TEXT

- Objectives, p. 512
- Interactive displays, pp. 512, 519, and 521
- Table 34-1. Penicillins, p. 514
- Table 34-2. Oral cephalosporins, p. 515
- Table 34-3. Parenteral cephalosporins, p. 516
- Nursing process, pp. 520
- Client teaching guidelines: Oral penicillins, p. 521
- Client teaching guidelines: Oral cephalosporins, p. 522
- Principles of therapy, p. 520
- Review and application exercises, pp. 527 and 528

TERMS AND CONCEPTS

Anaphylaxis
Beta-lactamase enzymes
Hypersensitivity

Penicillin-binding proteins
Cross-sensitivity

DRUG LIST

- Amoxicillin (Amoxil, Trimox)
- Ampicillin/Sulbactam (Unasyn)
- Dicloxacillin (Dynapen)
- Piperacillin (Pipracil)
- Penicillin G
- Penicillin V (Veetids)
- Cefaclor (Ceclor)
- Cefazolin (Kefzol, Ancef)
- Cefixime (Suprax)
- Ceftazidime (Fortaz)
- Ceftriaxone (Rocephin)
- Aztreonam (Azactam)
- Imipenem/Cilastatin (Primaxin)

■ Teaching Strategies

CLASSROOM

1. Show a transparency of the 4 types of beta-lactam drugs (transparency 29).

2. Show a transparency of the penicillin nucleus to demonstrate the beta-lactam chemical structure (transparency 28).

3. Prepare and show a transparency of the penicillins in the drug list, and remind students that generic names ending in "-cillin" are penicillins.

4. Discuss the mechanism of action of beta-lactamase inhibitors and the rationale for combining them with a penicillin.

5. Prepare and show a transparency of selected cephalosporins. Because there are several of these drugs in the first, second, and third generations, the instructor may wish to determine the ones most often used in local agencies and communities.

6. Note that the generic names of cephalosporins, except loracarbef (a synthetic drug), begin with "-cef" or "-ceph."

7. Discuss the role of cephalosporins in surgical chemoprophylaxis.

COLLABORATIVE ACTIVITIES FOR SMALL GROUPS

1. Assign groups to prepare a general teaching plan for oral penicillins; then compare their plans with a drug reference on an individual penicillin (amoxicillin is the most commonly used agent for ambulatory clients).

2. Write 2 copies of several drug names, and have half of students draw a drug name. Then, assign pairs of students to list the main client teaching points for the drug. Next, match 2 pairs with the same drug; ask them to compare their plans and indicate any differences. Ask that written work be signed by pair members and turned in.

3. Discuss and write responses to review and application exercises 6, 10, 11, and 12 (text, pp. 527 and 528). Some groups can be asked to report their findings to the entire class.

4. Discuss and write answers to the Critical Thinking Case Study (Study Guide, p. 113).

CLINICAL LABORATORY

1. For a group of clients, have students identify those who are receiving a penicillin (or the instructor can identify such clients from medication records) and discuss reasons for its use and drug effects in particular clients.

2. For clients who are receiving a penicillin/beta-lactamase inhibitor, ask students to identify the penicillin subgroup, the dose and route of administration, and a rationale for using the drug, the dose, and the route for a particular client.

3. For clients receiving a cephalosporin, have students review culture and susceptibility reports, the location of the infection or surgical procedure, and the specific drug; then, have students evaluate the appropriateness of the drug for the particular client.

4. For clients receiving an intravenous penicillin or cephalosporin, discuss how the drug is provided and intravenous fluids with which the drug is mixed.

5. For clients receiving a beta-lactam drug, ask students to assess for adverse effects and verbally report findings in a postclinical conference.

6. For a client newly started on an oral penicillin or cephalosporin, obtain an agency instruction sheet and discuss ways to individualize the instructions.

■ Critical Thinking Case Study

1. Ampicillin is a broad-spectrum, semisynthetic penicillin that is bactericidal for several types of gram-positive and gram-negative bacteria. It is effective in treating *Shigella* infections.

2. The route of choice depends on the seriousness of the infection. Normally this type of infection would be treated with oral antibiotics, but Mr. B. is an insulin-dependent diabetic. An infectious process could elevate his blood sugar. Because Mr. B. is also dehydrated, intravenous therapy is appropriate in his case.

3. Perform a complete assessment, including vital signs and respiratory assessment. A rash is a hypersensitivity reaction, and his physician should be notified.

CHAPTER 35

Aminoglycosides and Fluoroquinolones

MAJOR TOPICS

- Types of infections for which aminoglycosides are used
- Comparison with beta-lactam antibiotics
- Major adverse effects of aminoglycosides
- Fluoroquinolone uses and effects

QUICK REFERENCE GUIDE TO TEXT

- Objectives, p. 529
- Interactive displays, pp. 529 and 535
- Table 35-1. Aminoglycosides, p. 531
- Table 35-2. Fluoroquinolones, p. 533
- Nursing process, pp. 534 and 537
- Client teaching guidelines: Oral fluoroquinolones, p. 534
- Principles of therapy, p. 534
- Review and application exercises, p. 539

TERMS AND CONCEPTS

Audiometry
Nephrotoxicity
Ototoxicity

Peak and trough serum
drug levels
Postantibiotic effect

DRUG LIST

- Amikacin (Amikin)
- Ciprofloxacin (Cipro)
- Gentamicin (Garamycin)

■ Teaching Strategies

CLASSROOM

1. Lecture/discussion about uses and effects of aminoglycosides, according to objectives.

2. Emphasize gentamicin as the most commonly used aminoglycoside and amikacin as commonly used when gentamicin-resistant organisms develop.

3. Lecture/discussion about uses and effects of fluoroquinolones. Note that these drugs are contraindicated in children.

4. Point out that generic names of fluoroquinolones all end in "-oxacin."

5. Emphasize ciprofloxacin as a commonly used fluoroquinolone.

COLLABORATIVE ACTIVITIES FOR SMALL GROUPS

1. Discuss review and application exercises 4 through 10 (text, p. 539).

2. Discuss review and application exercises 12 through 14 (text, pp. 539 and 540).

CLINICAL LABORATORY

1. For a group of clients, identify those at risk of developing nephrotoxicity with aminoglycosides.

2. Have students participate in ensuring that blood for peak and trough drug levels is drawn at appropriate times.

3. For all patients receiving a systemic aminoglycoside, have students monitor serum drug levels and renal function tests (eg, blood urea nitrogen, serum creatinine) for abnormal values.

4. Have students measure fluid intake and urine output and provide other interventions to ensure that a client receiving a systemic aminoglycoside or a fluoroquinolone is well hydrated to preserve renal function and decrease risks of nephrotoxicity.

5. For a client who is receiving a fluoroquinolone, have students assess the reason for use and the client's response (ie, therapeutic and adverse effects).

■ Critical Thinking Case Study

1. Before initiating therapy, the client's renal status should be assessed. During treatment, the nurse should be observing for symptoms of nephrotoxicity, which include increased creatinine and BUN and decreased urinary output.

2. An acceptable urinary output is 30 mL/hr, but given the high incidence of renal toxicity associated with aminoglycoside use, you should also assess 24-hour intakes and outputs, vital signs, weight, and laboratory values. If there is a significant drop in output or another assessment is deviated, you should contact the physician.

3. There is an increased risk of nephrotoxicity with concurrent use of aminoglycosides and diuretics. Therefore, you need to check with the physician before you administer the antibiotic. Lasix should be administered slowly, and you should continue to assess the client's renal status.

CHAPTER 36

Tetracyclines, Sulfonamides, and Urinary Agents

MAJOR TOPICS

- Types of infections for which tetracyclines are used
- Contraindications to tetracycline use
- Uses of sulfonamides
- Drug therapy for urinary tract infections

QUICK REFERENCE GUIDE TO TEXT

- Objectives, p. 541
- Interactive displays, pp. 541, 547, and 550
- Table 36-1. Tetracyclines, p. 542
- Table 36-2. Sulfonamide preparations, p. 543
- Table 36-3. Miscellaneous drugs for UTI, p. 545
- Nursing process, pp. 548 and 549
- Client teaching guidelines: Oral tetracyclines, p. 548
- Client teaching guidelines: Oral sulfonamides, p. 549
- Principles of therapy, p. 549
- Review and application exercises, p. 553

TERMS AND CONCEPTS

Antianabolic effect	Crystalluria
Antimetabolite	Mineralization
Azotemia	

DRUG LIST

- Doxycycline (Vibramycin)
- Tetracycline (Sumycin)
- Trimethoprim/sulfamethoxazole (Bactrim)

■ Teaching Strategies

CLASSROOM

1. Tetracyclines are used infrequently in most clinical practice settings, and the instructor may wish to provide a handout summarizing main points rather than spending class time. Note that most standardized pharmacology tests include 1 or more items about food and drug interactions that decrease absorption of oral tetracyclines.

2. Discuss the reasons that sulfonamides are infrequently used for systemic infections.

COLLABORATIVE ACTIVITIES FOR SMALL GROUPS

1. Discuss review and application exercises (text, p. 553).

2. Discuss the Critical Thinking Case Study (study guide, p. 119).

3. Prepare a teaching plan for clients with a UTI; include interventions to heal the current UTI and prevent future occurrences.

CLINICAL LABORATORY

1. For clients receiving an oral tetracycline, have students assess knowledge about correct self-administration (ie, not taking the drug with certain foods and other drugs).

2. For a client receiving an intravenous tetracycline, check the venipuncture site at least twice daily for phlebitis.

3. For clients receiving a systemic sulfonamide, have students assess intake and output and renal function tests for abnormal values.

■ Critical Thinking Case Study

1. Assess her knowledge of tetracycline and be sure that she is not pregnant.

2. Discuss how and when to take the medication. Adverse effects should be discussed, specifically photosensitivity.

3. I would ask her whether she has been taking her medication every day on an empty stomach. I would also find out what her expectations were of the medication.

4. A sore throat may be indicative of thrush. After examining her throat and lymph nodes, I would decide whether a throat culture is warranted.

CHAPTER 37

Macrolides and Miscellaneous Antibacterials

MAJOR TOPICS

- Types of infections for which macrolides are used
- Interference of erythromycin with metabolism of other drugs
- Selected miscellaneous antibacterial drugs
- CDC guidelines for using vancomycin to prevent VRE

QUICK REFERENCE GUIDE TO TEXT

- Objectives, p. 554
- Interactive displays, pp. 554, 558, and 560
- Table 37-1. Macrolides, p. 556
- Nursing process, p. 558
- Client teaching guidelines: Macrolides, p. 559
- Principles of therapy, p. 559
- Review and application exercises, p. 564

TERMS AND CONCEPTS

Cytochrome P450 enzymes   Pseudomembranous colitis
Hepatotoxicity

DRUG LIST

- Azithromycin (Zithromax)
- Clarithromycin (Biaxin)
- Clindamycin (Cleocin)
- Erythromycin (Ery-Tab, Erythrocin)
- Metronidazole (Flagyl)
- Vancomycin (Vancocin)

■ Teaching Strategies

CLASSROOM

1. Discuss uses and effects of macrolide antibiotics.
2. Compare and contrast erythromycin and the newer macrolides.
3. Provide a written handout summarizing the main points about the miscellaneous drugs.
4. Discuss the reasons for restricting use of vancomycin.

COLLABORATIVE ACTIVITIES FOR SMALL GROUPS

1. Discuss the scenario regarding MRSA (text, p. 554).
2. Discuss review and application exercises 7 through 9 (text, p. 564).
3. Prepare a teaching plan for a client taking a newly prescribed macrolide.

CLINICAL LABORATORY

1. In a hospital or long-term care facility, the instructor can scan the medication administration record for clients receiving a macrolide; then, assign students to assess clients for therapeutic and adverse effects.
2. In outpatient settings, have students individualize an agency instruction sheet for a client with a newly prescribed macrolide.
3. For a client taking a miscellaneous drug, have a student assess the reason for use (including culture and susceptibility reports) and the client's response (ie, therapeutic and adverse effects).

4. For a group of clients, have students identify those at risk of developing pseudomembranous colitis and how they plan to assess for this condition.

5. In a hospital setting, ask a pharmacist, infectious disease physician, or infection control nurse about restrictions on the use of vancomycin.

■ Critical Thinking Case Study

1. The assessment would include breath sounds, chest X-ray, vital signs, and a sputum culture if he has a productive cough.

2. Mr. R. should rest and drink lots of fluids. He may be up walking to try and mobilize his secretions. He may use antipyretics to control his fever. Ideally, erythromycin should be taken on an empty stomach, but because it causes stomach upset it may be taken with food if necessary.

3. Ask her if he has tried the medication with food and if he has been able to keep anything down. Also, ask what her husband's pulse rate and temperature are and whether he has urinated and how much. If it is apparent that Mr. R. is dehydrated and unable to keep anything down, he should come to the office.

4. If Mr. R. is still vomiting after 2 days, ask the physician to change the medication.

CHAPTER 38

Drugs for Tuberculosis and *Mycobacterium avium* Complex (MAC) Disease

MAJOR TOPICS

- Characteristics of TB infections
- Risk factors for developing multidrug-resistant TB
- Drug therapy for TB

QUICK REFERENCE GUIDE TO TEXT

- Objectives, p. 565
- Interactive displays, pp. 565 and 572
- Table 38-1. Selected antitubercular drugs, p. 568
- Nursing process, pp. 570–572
- Client teaching guidelines: Isoniazid, rifampin, and pyrazinamide, p. 571
- Principles of therapy, p. 572
- Review and application exercises, p. 576

TERMS AND CONCEPTS

Directly observed therapy	Jaundice
Hepatitis	Peripheral neuritis

DRUG LIST

- Isoniazid (INH)
- Pyrazinamide
- Pyridoxine (vitamin B$_6$)
- Rifampin (Rifadin)

■ Teaching Strategies

CLASSROOM

1. Discuss patient teaching materials available from the local health department.

2. Ask a nurse in the TB clinic of the local health department to speak to the class about current recommendations for prevention and treatment of TB.

3. Ask students to list nursing interventions to promote compliance with drug therapy regimens. Write the list on a transparency or marker board. Ask students to evaluate each proposed intervention in terms of expected effectiveness, ease or difficulty with implementation, potential cost in money and time, and likely availability of sufficient state or local funds.

COLLABORATIVE ACTIVITIES FOR SMALL GROUPS

1. Discuss the client scenario (text, p. 565).

2. Ask students to "brainstorm" about (and list) possible ways to implement directly observed therapy for various populations (eg, rural, mentally ill, homeless). The instructor can then ask selected groups to report their findings, write suggestions on a marker board or transparency, and ask other groups if they agree, disagree, or have additions.

3. Assign 1 or 2 review and application exercises (text, p. 576) to each group, to be discussed with the entire class or written and turned in after the group activity.

4. Discuss the Critical Thinking Case Study (study guide, p. 125).

CLINICAL LABORATORY

1. Review agency policies and procedures regarding interventions to protect patients and health care providers from TB infection.

2. Ask a hospital infection control nurse to speak regarding management of patients with suspected or confirmed TB.

3. For hospitalized clients with suspected or known TB, have students review culture and susceptibility reports (if available), write or verbally discuss prescribed drug therapy, describe medical isolation procedures (eg, during postclinical conference), and discuss any violations of medical isolation procedures observed.

▪ Critical Thinking Case Study

1. You will need to take the medication for 1 year and have a yearly chest X-ray instead of a skin test.

2. These may be adverse reactions to the medication. You need to be seen by your physician, who will evaluate you and decide whether to discontinue the medication.

CHAPTER 39

Antiviral Drugs

MAJOR TOPICS

- Viruses and viral infections
- Types of antiviral drugs
- Uses and effects of antiviral drugs

QUICK REFERENCE GUIDE TO TEXT

TERMS AND CONCEPTS

Acquired immunodeficiency syndrome (AIDS)

Cytomegalovirus (CMV) retinitis

Genital herpes

Human immunodeficiency virus (HIV)

Immunocompromise

Retrovirus

DRUG LIST

- Acyclovir (Zovirax)
- Indinavir (Crixivan)
- Nevirapine (Viramune)
- Oseltamivir (Tamiflu)
- Saquinavir (Invirase)
- Zanamivir (Relenza)
- Zidovudine (Retrovir)

■ Teaching Strategies

CLASSROOM

1. Lecture/discussion regarding some ways viral infections and antiviral drug therapy differ from bacterial infections and antibacterial drug therapy. (This approach attempts to relate the unknown to the known, because students are likely to be more familiar with antibacterial drugs than with antiviral drugs.)

2. Emphasize those antiviral drugs that students are most likely to encounter in clinical practice.

3. Discuss types, uses, and effects of antiviral drugs for influenza, genital herpes, and HIV infection.

4. Show a transparency of Figure 39-1 (text, p. 586; transparency 30), to demonstrate the actions of anti-AIDS drugs.

5. With anti-AIDS drugs, discuss the rationale for combination drug therapy.

6. Have students obtain, read, and summarize a journal article related to HIV infection and its treatment. The instructor may require a computer

search for appropriate articles or list names of journals likely to contain such articles.

7. If feasible, ask a client with HIV infection or a health care provider who works with AIDS patients to speak to the class regarding the medical, psychosocial, and economic aspects of living with HIV infection.

8. Discuss interventions to preserve kidney function when nephrotoxic antiviral drugs are used.

COLLABORATIVE ACTIVITIES FOR SMALL GROUPS

1. Discuss the client scenario (text, p. 578).

2. Prepare a teaching plan for a client on newly prescribed oseltamivir or zanamivir for influenza infection.

3. Discuss review and application exercises (text, p. 598).

4. Discuss the Critical Thinking Case Study (study guide, p. 128).

CLINICAL LABORATORY

1. In an outpatient setting, have students provide verbal and written instructions to clients receiving an oral antiviral drug.

2. In a hospital setting, assign students to immunocompromised clients who are receiving an intravenous antiviral drug. Once they have had time and opportunity to assess clients, question them about the factors contributing to each client's immunocompromised status, the viral infection being treated, administration and adverse effects of the specific antiviral drug, and their planned interventions.

3. For hospitalized clients with HIV infection, discuss agency infection control procedures.

4. For a client with HIV infection, ask a student to interview the client about behaviors of nurses and other health care providers that the client finds helpful or desirable.

5. For hospitalized clients receiving a nephrotoxic antiviral drug, ask students to monitor BUN, serum creatinine, and intake and output for abnormal values.

6. Ask students to identify clients at high risk for influenza infection and discuss the need for annual influenza vaccination, if indicated.

■ Critical Thinking Case Study

1. This drug does not prevent transmission of the virus. Granulocytopenia and anemia can develop. The drug may need to be stopped temporarily until your bone marrow recovers.

2. Anxiety; Risk for Injury: Recurrent infections; Social Isolation.

3. The medication is administered parenterally, twice a day for 2 to 3 weeks. A maintenance dose is then given once a day for 5 or 7 days a week. The drug will improve your condition but not cure it.

4. Try to find out from him the location and amount of bleeding. If he is hemorrhaging, give him some suggestions to stop the bleeding and tell him to call 911. If you perceive that the situation is not serious, allow him time to express his feelings.

CHAPTER 40

Antifungal Drugs

MAJOR TOPICS

- Types of fungal infections
- Characteristics of antifungal drug therapy

QUICK REFERENCE GUIDE TO TEXT

- Objectives, p. 600
- Interactive displays, pp. 600, 606, and 608
- Table 40-1. Selected antifungal drugs, p. 604
- Box 40-1. Selected fungal infections, p. 601
- Nursing process, pp. 603 and 606
- Client teaching guidelines: Oral and topical antifungals, p. 607
- Principles of therapy, p. 606
- Review and application exercises, p. 612

TERMS AND CONCEPTS

Candidiasis   Mycoses
Dermatophytes

DRUG LIST

- Amphotericin B (Fungizone, Abelcet)
- Fluconazole (Diflucan)

■ Teaching Strategies

CLASSROOM

1. Lecture/discussion regarding some ways fungal infections and antifungal drug therapy differ from bacterial infections and antibacterial drug therapy. (This approach attempts to relate the unknown to the known, because students are likely to be more familiar with antibacterial drugs than with antifungal drugs.)

2. Emphasize those antifungal drugs that students are most likely to encounter in clinical practice.

COLLABORATIVE ACTIVITIES FOR SMALL GROUPS

1. Discuss the client scenario (text, p. 600).

2. Discuss review and application exercises (text, p. 612).

CLINICAL LABORATORY

1. Have students assess all clients receiving a systemic antibacterial drug for signs and symptoms of candidiasis.

2. In an outpatient setting, have students provide verbal and written instructions to clients receiving an oral or topical antifungal drug.

3. In a hospital setting, assign students to clients who are receiving an intravenous antifungal drug. Once they have had time and opportunity to assess clients, question them about reasons for using the prescribed drug and their planned interventions related to administering and observing effects of the drug.

■ Critical Thinking Case Study

1. One of the adverse effects of this drug is photosensitivity. If she is working in the sun, she is at risk for burning. To treat fungal infection of the nails, it is best that artificial nails not be applied to the area; it could jeopardize the healing process.

2. Eat regularly to avoid gastrointestinal upset, and apply sunscreen. Look out for the adverse effects, and notify a physician if you are experiencing any.

3. Knowledge Deficit; Risk for Injury: Related to Adverse Effects of Drugs; Risk for Noncompliance.

4. These are possibly symptoms of an adverse effect of the medication. Explain to the client that a complete examination should be performed before a decision is made to stop or change the medication.

CHAPTER 41

Antiparasitics

MAJOR TOPICS

- Protozoal and helminthic infestations
- Scabies and pediculosis
- Prevention and treatment of parasitic infestations

QUICK REFERENCE GUIDE TO TEXT

- Objectives, p. 614
- Interactive displays, pp. 614 and 623
- Table 41-1. Antiparasitic drugs, p. 618
- Box 41-1. Helminthic infections, p. 617
- Nursing process, pp. 622 and 623
- Client teaching guidelines: Antiparasitic drugs, p. 624
- Principles of therapy, p. 625
- Review and application exercises, p. 628

TERMS AND CONCEPTS

Amebicide	Pediculicide
Anthelmintic	Plasmodia
Giardiasis	Pneumocystosis
Larvae	

DRUG LIST

- Chloroquine (Aralen)
- Mebendazole (Vermox)
- Metronidazole (Flagyl)
- Permethrin (Nix, Elimite)

■ Teaching Strategies

CLASSROOM

1. Emphasize those parasitic disorders that students are likely to encounter.

2. Discuss environmental factors that promote parasitic diseases.

3. Ask a school nurse or pediatric nurse to speak to the class about the incidence and treatment of pinworm and lice infestations.

COLLABORATIVE ACTIVITIES FOR SMALL GROUPS

1. Discuss the scenario regarding head lice in a school (text, p. 614).

2. Discuss the review and application exercises (text, p. 628).

CLINICAL LABORATORY

1. For clients with parasitic infestations, have students teach them about preventing recurrences.

2. Assign students to spend a day with a school nurse or with a nurse at a local health department that provides information and prophylactic drugs to overseas travelers.

3. In home care settings, assess for environmental and personal risk factors for the development of parasitic disorders and intervene as indicated.

DRUGS AFFECTING HEMATOPOIESIS AND THE IMMUNE SYSTEM

CHAPTER 42

Physiology of the Hematopoietic and Immune Systems

MAJOR TOPICS

- Body defense mechanisms
- Immunity
- Immune cells
- Immune disorders

QUICK REFERENCE GUIDE TO TEXT

TERMS AND CONCEPTS

Acquired immunity	Hematopoiesis
Antibody	Immunoglobulins
Antigen	Innate or natural immunity
Complement	Macrophage
Cytokines	Phagocytosis

■ Teaching Strategies

CLASSROOM

1. Assign students to read the chapter and write definitions of unfamiliar terms before class.

2. Lecture/discussion, using objectives as a guide. Emphasize that this content is vital to understanding immune functions and treatment of immune disorders.

3. Show a transparency of Figure 42-1, Normal hematopoiesis and immune cell development (text, p. 636; transparency 31).

4. Discuss the review and application exercises (text, p. 640).

CLINICAL LABORATORY

1. Assign students to care for clients with an immune disorder.

2. Ask students to list and evaluate clients' white blood cell counts and differential reports for indications of increased susceptibility to infection.

CHAPTER 43

Immunizing Agents

MAJOR TOPICS

- Active immunity
- Passive immunity

QUICK REFERENCE GUIDE TO TEXT

- Objectives, p. 641
- Interactive displays, pp. 641 and 653
- Table 43-1. Vaccines and toxoids for active immunity, p. 642
- Table 43-2. Immune serums and antitoxins for passive immunity, p. 650
- Box 43-1. Standards for pediatric immunization practices, p. 654
- Nursing process, pp. 650 and 652
- Client teaching guidelines: Immunizations, p. 653
- Principles of therapy, p. 653
- Review and application exercises, p. 658

TERMS AND CONCEPTS

Active immunity	Toxoid
Immunization	Vaccine
Passive immunity	

DRUG LIST

- Diphtheria-tetanus-pertussis vaccine (DTwP and DTaP)
- DTwP and *Haemophilus influnzae* type b (HIB) combined (Tetramune)
- HIB vaccine (HibTITER, PedvaxHIB, ProHIBiT)
- Hepatitis B vaccine, recombinant (Recombivax HB, Engerix-B)
- Pneumococcal vaccine (Pneumovax 23)

■ Teaching Strategies

CLASSROOM

1. Ask students about their attitudes and experiences in relation to immunizations.
2. Review routine immunization of young children or provide a written handout summarizing current recommendations.
3. Discuss desirability and practicality of standards for pediatric immunizations.

COLLABORATIVE ACTIVITIES FOR SMALL GROUPS

1. Discuss the infant immunization scenario (text, p. 641).
2. "Brainstorm" and list ways to teach parents and caregivers to promote immunizations of children. The instructor may then list group-generated ideas on a transparency or marker board and discuss them with the entire class.
3. Discuss the Critical Thinking Case Study (study guide, p. 139).

CLINICAL LABORATORY

1. Have students participate in administering immunizations in a physician's office, outpatient clinic, or long-term care facility.

2. Have students participate in teaching community groups (eg, schoolchildren, parents, senior citizens) about immunizations.

3. Have students evaluate the immunization status of assigned clients and explore mechanisms for obtaining needed ones.

4. Discuss possible approaches to an adult client with chronic lung disease who refuses to take influenza vaccine.

■ Critical Thinking Case Study

1. Ask the mother what kind of a reaction the infant had and how she treated it.

2. She will require proof of immunizations or a waiver before she can be admitted to school. She will be exposed to childhood illnesses, and if she is unimmunized and contracts an illness she could be extremely ill and be out of school for a significant amount of time.

3. Assess her for a fever and any respiratory problems.

4. It is not uncommon for children to have slight swelling at the injection site for a day or two. Give her some Tylenol to help with the discomfort. You can also give her a warm bath or apply a warm compress.

CHAPTER 44

Hematopoietic and Immunostimulant Drugs

MAJOR TOPICS

- Colony-stimulating factors
- Hematopoietic growth factors
- Interferons
- Interleukins

QUICK REFERENCE GUIDE TO TEXT

- Objectives, p. 659
- Interactive displays, pp. 659 and 666
- Table 44-1. Hematopoietic and immunostimulant agents, p. 660
- Nursing process, pp. 664 and 665
- Client teaching guidelines: Blood cell and immune system stimulants, p. 665
- Principles of therapy, p. 665
- Review and application exercises, p. 671

TERMS AND CONCEPTS

Colony-stimulating factors (CSFs)	Immunostimulant
Erythropoietin	Immunotherapy
Immunocompetence	Myelosuppression
Immunodeficiency	Neutropenia

DRUG LIST

- Epoetin alfa (Epogen)
- Filgrastim (Neupogen)
- Interferon alfa-2a (Roferon-A)
- Interferon beta-1b (Betaseron)

■ Teaching Strategies

CLASSROOM

1. Because this content is relatively complex, it is especially important that students prepare for class. Assignments may include reading the chapter in the text, writing descriptions of unfamiliar terms, looking up the listed drugs, and reviewing immune system physiology (see Chap. 42 or a physiology text).

2. Lecture/discussion regarding recent developments in this aspect of immunotherapy.

3. Ask students about their experiences with patients likely to receive these drugs (eg, those with bone marrow transplants or cancer).

COLLABORATIVE ACTIVITIES FOR SMALL GROUPS

1. Prepare a teaching plan for a client starting erythropoietin injections three times weekly.

2. Discuss the Critical Thinking Case Study (study guide, p. 142).

CLINICAL LABORATORY

1. Assign students to care for clients with a bone marrow transplant, cancer chemotherapy, or AIDS or another immunodeficiency disorder. Ask students to identify potential benefits of immunostimulant drug therapy.

2. Have students administer the listed drugs when opportunities arise.

3. For clients receiving any one of the listed drugs, have students assess for therapeutic and adverse effects.

■ Critical Thinking Case Study

1. CBC and platelet counts will be checked frequently. Avoid crowds, because you are at risk for infection. Nausea and vomiting can occur. Eat small, frequent meals. Report fever, chills, sore throat, weakness, and difficulty breathing.

2. The client's vital signs, heart sounds, lung sounds, weight, CBC with differential, and platelet count will be monitored.

3. We do not know at this time whether your graft has been successful. We will be monitoring you closely to evaluate the effectiveness of the medication and your response to it.

CHAPTER 45

Immunosuppressants

MAJOR TOPICS

- Autoimmune disorders
- Tissue and organ transplantation

QUICK REFERENCE GUIDE TO TEXT

- Objectives, p. 673
- Interactive displays, pp. 673 and 687
- Table 45-1. Immunosuppressants, p. 676
- Figure 45-1. Sites of action of immunosuppressants, p. 675
- Nursing process, pp. 681–683
- Client teaching guidelines: Immunosuppressant drugs, p. 684
- Principles of therapy, p. 683
- Review and application exercises, p. 695

TERMS AND CONCEPTS

Autoimmune disorders	Graft-versus-host disease
Cytotoxic	Immunosuppression
Graft rejection reactions	

DRUG LIST

- Azathioprine (Imuran)
- Cyclosporine (Sandimmune)
- Muromonab-CD3 (Orthoclone OKT3)
- Prednisone
- Tacrolimus (FK-506) (Prograf)

■ Teaching Strategies

CLASSROOM

1. Ask students about their previous experiences, if any, with clients undergoing transplantation or receiving immunosuppressant drug therapy.

2. Lecture/discussion regarding characteristics, indications for use, adverse effects, and nursing process implications of selected drugs.

3. Show a transparency of Figure 45-1 (text, p. 675; transparency 32).

4. Discuss the high risks of infection associated with immunosuppressant drug therapy and nursing interventions to prevent infection.

COLLABORATIVE ACTIVITIES FOR SMALL GROUPS

1. Prepare a teaching plan for a client being started on immunosuppressant drug therapy.

2. Discuss the review and application exercises (text, p. 695).

3. Discuss the Critical Thinking Case Study (study guide, p. 144).

CLINICAL LABORATORY

1. For a client receiving an immunosuppressant drug, have students check laboratory reports to monitor therapeutic and adverse drug effects (eg, BUN and serum creatinine as indicators of renal function in clients receiving cyclosporine).

2. Assign students to administer immunosuppressant drugs to transplantation patients and monitor drug effects.

3. Interview a client who has been receiving an immunosuppressant drug for a while to determine drug effects, usual practices to prevent infection and their success rate, the client's perceptions of helpful and nonhelpful behaviors of health care providers, and suggestions for nursing students caring for similar clients.

■ Critical Thinking Case Study

1. Vital signs will be evaluated. Changes could indicate fluid overload or infection. Intake and output and daily weight will be monitored carefully, because organ rejection can be heralded by decreased urinary output and weight gain. Elevations in serum creatinine, BUN, and potassium levels would indicate kidney failure.

2. The adverse effects of prednisone include fluid retention, elevated blood glucose concentration, electrolyte imbalances, and increased risk of infection. Persons receiving cyclosporine should be observed for symptoms of nephrotoxicity.

3. You will take immunosuppressive drugs the rest of your life, and the doses may need to be adjusted from time to time. You will be at increased risk for infection.

4. At this point, we do not know whether you will lose your kidney. It is not uncommon for persons who have undergone transplantation to have dialysis. Right now we will watch the situation very carefully. Your medication may need to be adjusted, and you may need to be dialyzed several times before your kidney starts functioning.

DRUGS AFFECTING THE RESPIRATORY SYSTEM

CHAPTER 46

Physiology of the Respiratory System

MAJOR TOPICS

- Structure and function of respiratory tract
- Normal respiration
- Common respiratory disorders for which drug therapy is often needed

QUICK REFERENCE GUIDE TO TEXT

- Objectives, p. 699
- Review and application exercises, p. 702

TERMS AND CONCEPTS

Anoxia	Oxygenation
Hypoxemia	Ventilation
Hypoxia	

■ Teaching Strategies

CLASSROOM

1. Lecture/discussion, using the objectives as an outline.
2. Suggest that students review content in a physiology text, if desired.

CLINICAL LABORATORY

1. Have students assess each assigned client for actual or potential interferences in respiratory functions (eg, excessive secretions).
2. For hospitalized clients, have students list laboratory results (eg, arterial blood gases, hemoglobin) and other diagnostic test reports of respiratory function and analyze them in terms of nursing process implications.

CHAPTER 47

Bronchodilating and Other Antiasthmatic Drugs

MAJOR TOPICS

- Asthma
- Chronic obstructive pulmonary disease
- Types of bronchodilating medications
- Use of antiasthmatic medications in special populations

QUICK REFERENCE GUIDE TO TEXT

- Objectives, p. 703
- Interactive displays, pp. 703, 711, and 712
- Table 47-1. Bronchodilating drugs, p. 705
- Table 47-2. Anti-inflammatory antiasthmatic drugs, p. 706
- Nursing process, pp. 708 and 709
- Client teaching guidelines: Antiasthmatic drugs, p. 710
- Principles of therapy, p. 711
- Review and application exercises, p. 716

TERMS AND CONCEPTS

Aerosol	Cyanosis
Bronchoconstriction	Nebulization
Bronchodilation	Status asthmaticus
Bronchospasm	Wheezing

DRUG LIST

- Albuterol (Proventil, Ventolin)
- Beclomethasone (Vanceril)
- Cromolyn (Intal)
- Epinephrine (Adrenalin)
- Ipratropium (Atrovent)
- Salmeterol (Serevent)
- Theophylline (Theo-Dur, aminophylline, others)
- Zafirlukast (Accolate)

■ Teaching Strategies

CLASSROOM

1. Lecture/discussion, using the objectives as an outline.
2. Show a transparency of the main pathophysiologic characteristics of asthma (transparency 33) and relate these characteristics to the types of drugs used for treatment.
3. Show a transparency of types of antiasthmatic drugs (transparency 34).
4. Ask students about their experiences with clients receiving medications via oral inhalation.

COLLABORATIVE ACTIVITIES FOR SMALL GROUPS

1. List and discuss the main differences between antiasthmatic drug therapy in children and that in older adults.
2. Discuss use of antiasthmatic drugs in clients with renal or hepatic impairment or critical illness.
3. Prepare a teaching plan for a hospitalized client being discharged on zafirlukast twice daily and albuterol oral inhalation PRN.
4. Discuss the review and application exercises (text, p. 716).

CLINICAL LABORATORY

1. For clients with asthma or other bronchoconstrictive disorders, assign students to assess respiration; administer bronchodilating drugs by oral, inhalation, or intravenous routes; and observe for therapeutic and adverse effects of the drugs.

2. For students assigned to clients with asthma or other bronchoconstrictive disorders, question the students about assessment data, nursing diagnoses, goals, and planned interventions and evaluations.

3. Ask students to report serum theophylline levels and to describe how they will use the information in their nursing care.

4. Have students teach clients about antiasthmatic medications, especially correct use of drugs for acute asthma attacks.

■ Critical Thinking Case Study

1. It would be helpful to know how Jenny has been treating her cold. You should ask whether she has taken any OTC medication, because some products contain aspirin, which could have precipitated the attack. It would also be helpful to know how she has been using her inhaler, and whether she used the inhaler before exercising, because overuse can cause bronchoconstriction.

2. Accolate decreases inflammation and relieves dyspnea. Solu-Medrol has an anti-inflammatory effect that decreases the swelling in the airways.

3. Headaches can occur with the administration of Accolate. You should tell Jenny that it is an expected side effect but that you will continue to assess her condition on a regular basis.

4. You need to assess for side effects of the medication in addition to monitoring her respiratory status.

CHAPTER 48

Antihistamines

MAJOR TOPICS

- Sources and effects of histamine
- Types of histamine receptors
- Hypersensitivity reactions
- Effects of histamine$_1$ receptor antagonists

QUICK REFERENCE GUIDE TO TEXT

- Objectives, p. 717
- Interactive displays, pp. 717, 724, and 726
- Table 48-1. Commonly used antihistamines, p. 721
- Figure 48-1. Development of allergic rhinitis, p. 719
- Figure 48-2. Action of antihistamines, p. 723
- Nursing process, pp. 724 and 725
- Client teaching guidelines: Antihistamines, p. 725
- Principles of therapy, p. 726
- Review and application exercises, p. 729

TERMS AND CONCEPTS

Allergic rhinitis	Pruritus
Histamine	Sedation

DRUG LIST

- Cetirizine (Zyrtec)
- Diphenhydramine (Benadryl)
- Fexofenadine (Allegra)
- Loratidine (Claritin)

■ Teaching Strategies

CLASSROOM

1. Describe effects of histamine on body tissues; show a transparency of Figure 48-1 (text, p. 721; transparency 35).

2. Discuss actions of antihistamines, using a transparency of Figure 48-2 (text, p. 723; transparency 36).

3. Ask students about their personal use of antihistamines (eg, which ones they take, when they take them, how the drugs affect them in terms of their activities of daily living).

4. Discuss the use of antihistamines in special populations.

CLINICAL LABORATORY

1. For hospitalized clients receiving diphenhydramine for sleep, have students assess for anticholinergic effects and excessive sedation.

2. For hospitalized clients receiving an antihistamine, have students interview the clients about therapeutic and adverse effects.

■ Critical Thinking Case Study

1. Antivert was ordered to control your dizziness. Adverse effects include drowsiness, confusion, dry mouth, and anorexia.

2. A calm, stress-free environment may help you avoid or lessen the effects of an attack of vertigo.

CHAPTER 49

Nasal Decongestants, Antitussives, Mucolytics, and Cold Remedies

MAJOR TOPICS

- Signs and symptoms of respiratory disorders
- Types of drugs used to relieve common signs and symptoms
- Ingredients in multisymptom cold remedies

QUICK REFERENCE GUIDE TO TEXT

- Objectives, p. 730
- Interactive displays, pp. 730, 732, and 733
- Table 49-1. Nasal decongestants, antitussives, and expectorants, p. 734
- Table 49-2. Nonprescription cold, cough, and sinus remedies, p. 735
- Nursing process, p. 733
- Client teaching guidelines: Nasal decongestants, antitussives, and multi-ingredient cold remedies, p. 736
- Principles of therapy, p. 734
- Review and application exercises, p. 739

TERMS AND CONCEPTS

Antitussive	Expectorant
Decongestant	Mucolytic

DRUG LIST

- Dextromethorphan (Benylin DM, others)
- Phenylephrine (Neo-Synephrine)
- Phenylpropanolamine
- Pseudoephedrine (Sudafed)

■ Teaching Strategies

CLASSROOM

1. Lecture/discussion, using the objectives as a guide. Little class time may be needed, because most students are likely to be familiar with these drugs from personal use.

2. Discuss the review and application exercises (text, p. 739).

COLLABORATIVE ACTIVITIES FOR SMALL GROUPS

1. The instructor can ask students (during the previous class) to bring containers of multi-ingredient OTC cold remedies or provide copies of drug labels. Then, ask each group to analyze one or more products to answer the following questions:
   a. What are the active ingredients?
   b. What is the classification of each active ingredient?
   c. Is the amount of each active ingredient contained in the recommended dose therapeutic?
   d. Who should *not* take the product?
   e. Would you take this product yourself or recommend it for family and friends? Why or why not?

2. Discuss the scenario regarding an infant with a cold, (text, p. 730).

3. Discuss the review and application exercises (text, p. 739) if not previously discussed in class.

CLINICAL LABORATORY

1. When assessing assigned clients, have students ask whether they use OTC cold remedies. If so, obtain the name of the product, the amount and frequency

of use, and the client's perception of therapeutic or adverse effects. Then, use a drug reference to analyze the ingredients and the instructions for use to determine whether the particular client can safely continue to use the product.

2. For clients with a disease process or other drug therapy that is likely to interact adversely with an OTC cold remedy, have students teach about products to avoid or to use cautiously and advise clients to always read the label before using the product.

■ Critical Thinking Case Study

1. Guaifenesin and Mucomyst are expectorants. Mr. Z. should increase his fluid intake; turn, cough, and deep breathe (TCDB); and ambulate, if possible, to mobilize his secretions. Mucomyst has an unpleasant taste, so he will want to rinse his mouth after using it. Prednisone is used for short periods to decrease inflammation. It can cause gastrointestinal bleeding, so antacids may be administered with it.

2. Breath sounds will be assessed every shift; congestion should improve daily. Vital signs will be assessed; his temperature should go down. Laboratory values will also be monitored for blood glucose levels, electrolytes, and CBC count.

3. Encourage him to TCDB and ambulate if possible. Offer him fluids at regular intervals.

4. The nausea could be related to the antibiotics. If he is not vomiting and is able to tolerate the nausea, nothing may be done. If the nausea is problematic, an antiemetic may be administered or the antibiotic may be changed.

5. Make sure that you get adequate exercise and rest. Increase your fluid intake and eat a well-balanced diet.

DRUGS AFFECTING THE CARDIOVASCULAR SYSTEM

CHAPTER 50

Physiology of the Cardiovascular System

MAJOR TOPICS

- Structure and function of the heart, blood vessels, and blood
- Endothelial factors in cardiovascular functioning
- Overview of cardiovascular disorders usually treated with drugs

QUICK REFERENCE GUIDE TO TEXT

- Objectives, p. 743
- Table 50-1. Endothelial mediators, p. 745
- Review and application exercises, p. 747

TERMS AND CONCEPTS

Arterioles	Nitric oxide
Atria	Perfusion
Endothelium	Procoagulant
Myocardium	Ventricles

■ Teaching Strategies

CLASSROOM

1. Lecture/discussion, using the objectives as an outline.
2. Discuss and refer to Table 50-1 (text, p. 745) to emphasize the importance of endothelial factors in regulating cardiovascular functions.
3. Assign students to study the chapter and write out answers to objectives.
4. Assign students to review content in a recent physiology text.

CLINICAL LABORATORY

1. Have students assess each assigned client for actual or potential cardiovascular disorders.
2. For hospitalized clients, have students check apical and radial pulses, blood pressure, ECG tracings, laboratory reports, other diagnostic test reports, and prescribed drugs. Then, have them analyze data in relation to possible cardiovascular disorders and nursing process implications.

CHAPTER 51

Drug Therapy of Heart Failure

MAJOR TOPICS

- Causes and clinical manifestations of heart failure
- Endothelial dysfunction in heart failure
- Types of drugs used to treat heart failure
- Effects of digoxin
- Management of digoxin toxicity

QUICK REFERENCE GUIDE TO TEXT

- Objectives, p. 748
- Interactive displays, pp. 748 and 753
- Box 51-1. New York Heart Association classification of patients with heart failure, p. 749
- Box 51-2. Drugs used to treat heart failure, p. 750
- Nursing process, pp. 753–755
- Client teaching guidelines: Digoxin, p. 755
- Principles of therapy, p. 756
- Review and application exercises, p. 763

TERMS AND CONCEPTS

Arrhythmia
Atrial fibrillation
Bradycardia
Cardiac output

Cardiotonic
Compensatory mechanisms
Digitalization
Inotropic

DRUG LIST

- Digoxin (Lanoxin)
- Digoxin immune Fab (Digibind, Digidote)

■ Teaching Strategies

CLASSROOM

1. Lecture/discussion, using the objectives as an outline.

2. Emphasize digoxin as a commonly prescribed drug that is likely to be encountered in any clinical setting.

3. Ask students to share their experiences and perceptions if they have had clients or family members who were taking digoxin.

COLLABORATIVE ACTIVITIES FOR SMALL GROUPS

1. As a class presentation, have 2 groups of students debate the desirability of discontinuing digoxin when possible.

2. Have students write answers to the review and application exercises (text, p. 763), then discuss them in class.

3. Discuss the precautions needed when digoxin is given to older adults and to people with impaired renal function.

4. Discuss the Critical Thinking Case Study (study guide, p. 163).

CLINICAL LABORATORY

1. For clients with CHF, have students assess for edema, fatigue, and respiratory distress.

2. For clients receiving digoxin, question students about the reason for its use and the drug effects.

3. For clients receiving digoxin, have students assess, verbalize, and record the rate and quality of apical and radial pulses.

4. For clients with atrial fibrillation and digoxin therapy, have students analyze 12-lead ECGs or cardiac monitoring strips for drug effects.

5. For clients receiving digoxin, ask students to explain why it is important to monitor for hypokalemia and what they will do if it occurs.

■ Critical Thinking Case Study

1. When a person is being digitalized, a larger than standard dose is administered in 2–3 equal doses. The physician will use M.'s weight to calculate the appropriate dose for M. M.'s pulse rate will drop once she is digitalized. Her heart will beat slower and more efficiently; therefore, the symptoms of heart failure should improve. Her urinary output may also increase because of the increased perfusion to her kidneys.

2. The adverse effects of digoxin include arrhythmias, anorexia, nausea, vomiting, headache, drowsiness, confusion, and visual disturbances. The symptoms of digoxin toxicity are vague and could be misinterpreted as flu symptoms; therefore, it is important for M.'s mother to check M.'s pulse and to contact the physician if M. has a concurrent pulse change along with other symptoms.

3. Drugs that decrease the effects of digoxin include antacids, cholestyramine, colestipol, laxatives, oral aminoglycosides, barbiturates, and phenytoin. Drugs that increase the effect of digoxin include adrenergic drugs, anticholinergic drugs, calcium preparations, quinidine, verapamil, and nifedipine.

4. The physician has ordered daily measurements of digoxin concentration to determine whether a therapeutic level has been reached. He is also evaluating M.'s electrolytes (K^+, Ca^{++}, Mg^{++}), because deviations in those electrolytes can potentiate digoxin toxicity.

5. Blood studies help establish whether medications are being administered. The symptoms of heart failure should improve if the treatment plan is followed.

6. Three nursing diagnoses that would be appropriate for M. are Altered Tissue Perfusion related to decreased cardiac output, Activity Intolerance related to decreased cardiac output, and Impaired Gas Exchange related to venous congestion and fluid accumulation.

CHAPTER 52

Antiarrhythmic Drugs

MAJOR TOPICS

- Normal cardiac conduction
- Types of arrhythmias
- Types of antiarrhythmic drugs
- Toxicity of antiarrhythmic drugs

QUICK REFERENCE GUIDE TO TEXT

- Objectives, p. 764
- Interactive displays, pp. 764 and 766
- Table 52-1. Antiarrhythmic drugs, p. 768
- Box 52-1. Types of arrhythmias, p. 767
- Figure 52-1. Cardiac conduction system, p. 765
- Figure 52-2. Reentry excitation of arrhythmias, p. 766
- Nursing process, pp. 773 and 774
- Client teaching guidelines: Antiarrhythmic drugs, p. 774
- Principles of therapy, p. 775
- Review and application exercises, p. 781

TERMS AND CONCEPTS

Arrhythmogenic	Dysrhythmia
Automaticity	Ectopic focus
Bradyarrhythmia	Refractory period
Cardiac depressants	Tachyarrhythmia

DRUG LIST

- Quinidine
- Lidocaine (Xylocaine)

■ Teaching Strategies

CLASSROOM

1. Lecture/discussion, using the objectives as an outline.
2. Show a transparency of Figure 52-1 (text, p. 765; transparency 37) to review the cardiac conduction system.
3. Show a transparency of Figure 52-2 (text, p. 766; transparency 38).
4. Ask a nurse who works in a coronary care unit to speak to the class about arrhythmias that commonly occur after myocardial infarction and how they may be prevented, recognized, or treated.

COLLABORATIVE ACTIVITIES FOR SMALL GROUPS

1. Prepare a general teaching plan for an adult client who is being started on an antiarrhythmic drug.
2. Discuss the Critical Thinking Case Study (study guide, p. 169).

CLINICAL LABORATORY

1. Have students compare ECG tracings (from continuous cardiac monitoring or 12-lead ECGs) for a client with an arrhythmia before and after administration of antiarrhythmic drugs.
2. Assign students to care for clients on telemetry units. Ask students to correlate their clinical observations (eg, vital signs, skin color and temperature, level of consciousness, overall status) with the clients' ECG tracings, antiarrhythmic medications, and other objective indicators of cardiovascular functioning.

3. Demonstrate a continuous intravenous lidocaine drip in an emergency or intensive care setting; discuss drug concentration, regulation of flow rate, and how to monitor the client's response.

■ Critical Thinking Case Study

1. The usual bolus does of lidocaine is 1–2 mg/kg, not to exceed 100 mg. If the physician uses Mr. J's weight to determine the dosage, he will order between 50 and 100 mg initially, followed by a continuous infusion. The continuous infusion is usually started at 1–2 mg/min and increased gradually until the PVCs are controlled. Lidocaine is always infused at the lowest possible rate to prevent toxic side effects.

2. If the present dose of lidocaine is not effective, it can be increased to a maximum of 4 mg/min. Mr. J should be observed for drowsiness, paresthesias, muscle twitching, convulsions, urticaria, edema, and anaphylaxis. Adverse reactions are more likely to occur at the higher dose. If Mr. J's PVCs are still not controlled, the physician should be notified. The physician has the option of ordering a Pronestyl or a Bretylium drip to control the PVCs.

3. Mr. J's ECG shows first-degree heart block. The physician should be contacted. The medication may be dispensed to control cardiac irritability, and the pulse and blood pressure and PR interval should be monitored at regular intervals.

4. After a heart attack, it is normal for people to experience a lack of energy for 4–6 weeks. The ability to climb two flights of stairs without becoming short of breath is a good indication that one has enough energy for sexual intercourse. Antiarrhythmic/antihypertensive medications, such as propranolol (Inderal), sometimes have an effect on sexual performance. If you experience a problem, contact your physician.

CHAPTER 53

Antianginal Drugs

MAJOR TOPICS

- Characteristics and types of angina pectoris
- Endothelial dysfunction and atherosclerosis
- Types of antianginal drugs
- Nitrates and calcium channel blockers

QUICK REFERENCE GUIDE TO TEXT

TERMS AND CONCEPTS

Angina pectoris	Hypoxia
Coronary atherosclerosis	Myocardial infarction
Hypoxemia	Myocardial ischemia

DRUG LIST

- Amlodipine (Norvasc)
- Diltiazem (Cardizem)
- Isosorbide mononitrate (Imdur)
- Nifedipine (Procardia, Adalat)
- Nitroglycerin (Nitro-Dur, Nitrostat)
- Verapamil (Calan)

■ Teaching Strategies

CLASSROOM

1. Lecture/discussion, using the objectives as an outline.

2. Differentiate onset and duration of action with various forms of nitroglycerin (eg, sublingual tablet, skin patch, intravenous infusion).

3. Compare antianginal effects of nitrates and beta blockers (transparency 39).

4. Coach and question students through a scenario in which a client with angina pectoris complains of chest pain. Include assessment needs, administration of sublingual nitroglycerin, observation of response, and teaching to prevent or manage future attacks.

5. Prepare and show a transparency of selected calcium channel blockers (transparency 40), such as verapamil as the first, nifedipine as the prototype of the dihydropyridine group (whose generic names end in "-dipine"), and 1 or 2 others that are commonly used in local clinical practice agencies.

6. Show a transparency of Figure 53-1 (text, p. 788; transparency 41) to demonstrate the mechanism of action for calcium channel blockers.

7. Show a transparency of cardiovascular indications for use of calcium channel blockers (transparency 42).

COLLABORATIVE ACTIVITIES FOR SMALL GROUPS

1. Prepare a teaching plan for a client beginning nitrate therapy.

2. Prepare a teaching plan for a client beginning a calcium channel blocker.

3. Discuss the Critical Thinking Case Study (study guide, p. 173).

CLINICAL LABORATORY

1. For clients receiving sublingual nitroglycerin, have students ensure that an adequate supply is available within the client's reach.

2. Have a student (or the instructor) interview a client who takes sublingual nitroglycerin as needed regarding how often the drug is used, how many tablets are taken and how close together, whether relief is obtained, how long it usually takes to obtain relief, whether dizziness or headache occurs, and so forth. This information is helpful in teaching other clients who are just starting to use sublingual nitroglycerin.

3. For a client who experiences acute angina while being cared for by a student, have the student assess vital signs, activities at onset of chest pain, and interventions that relieve pain.

4. For clients with cardiovascular disease, list the ordered drugs, show the list to students, and ask them to identify any antianginal drugs.

5. Have students locate and read agency instruction sheets regarding nitrates and calcium channel blockers.

■ Critical Thinking Case Study

1. Mr. D.'s vital signs will be checked every 15 minutes. Tachycardia and hypotension are 2 common adverse effects of nitroglycerin. Mr. D. must be watched closely, because hypotension can decrease blood supply to the coronary arteries, aggravating angina or precipitating a myocardial infarction. Mr. D.'s ECG will be monitored continuously, and a complete head-to-toe assessment will be performed once the chest pain subsides, including an evaluation of his heart sounds.

2. Diltiazem reportedly has the fewest adverse effects of all the calcium channel blockers; it is effective in treating angina and also lowers blood pressure. Because Mr. D experienced undesirable side effects from beta-adrenergic blockers, it is better to avoid the beta-adrenergic blocker category of drugs.

3. Headache and dizziness are encountered occasionally along with weakness. Mr. D.'s ECG should be monitored, because bradycardia and first-degree AV block can occur.

4. Persons taking long-acting nitrates on a regular schedule can develop a tolerance. Many physicians now order long-acting nitrates for 16 hours daily to prevent the development of tolerance in their clients. The adverse effects of nitroglycerin include hypotension, dizziness, and headache. These symptoms can be increased when another antianginal agent is given concurrently.

CHAPTER 54

Drugs Used in Hypotension and Shock

MAJOR TOPICS

- Types of shock
- Types of antishock drugs

QUICK REFERENCE GUIDE TO TEXT

- Objectives, p. 798
- Interactive displays, pp. 798, 802, and 803
- Table 54-1. Types of shock, p. 799
- Table 54-2. Drugs used for shock and hypotension, p. 800
- Nursing process, pp. 802 and 803
- Principles of therapy, p. 803
- Review and application exercises, p. 807

TERMS AND CONCEPTS

Alpha-adrenergic effects
Beta-adrenergic effects
Cardiogenic shock
Catecholamine
Hypovolemic shock

Neurogenic shock
Perfusion
Vasodilation
Vasopressor

DRUG LIST

- Dobutamine (Dobutrex)
- Dopamine (Intropin)
- Epinephrine (Adrenalin)
- Norepinephrine (Levophed)

■ Teaching Strategies

CLASSROOM

1. Lecture/discussion on types of shock (transparency 43).

2. Discuss the recognition and treatment of anaphylactic or hypovolemic shock. Emphasize that these emergencies may occur in any setting.

COLLABORATIVE ACTIVITIES FOR SMALL GROUPS

1. Discuss the review and application exercises (text, p. 807).

2. Discuss the Critical Thinking Case Study (study guide, p. 175).

CLINICAL LABORATORY

1. For a group of clients, have students identify those with risk factors for development of hypotension and shock.

2. Ask students to locate emergency drugs and supplies that would be needed for a patient in shock.

3. Role-play or conduct a "mock" emergency or rehearsal in which a student finds a client in shock and proceeds with appropriate interventions such as checking vital signs, skin color and temperature, and level of consciousness; calling a physician; bringing emergency drugs and other equipment to the client's location; and so forth.

■ Critical Thinking Case Study

1. Mr. B. weighs 100 kg; therefore, he should receive between 200 and 500 μg/min. You will assess Mr. B. for decreases in blood pressure, heart rate, urine output, skin temperature, and level of consciousness; all of these symptoms are commonly seen in shock and are the result of inadequate perfusion. The severity of the symptoms determines the course of action.

2. At moderate doses, dopamine increases heart rate, myocardial contractility, and blood pressure. Dobutamine increases the force of myocardial contraction and also increases blood pressure when larger doses are given, but it should not induce or contribute to tachycardia, which can increase oxygen demand. The physician is hoping to improve tissue perfusion. If the kidneys are adequately perfused, Mr. B.'s urinary output should increase.

3. Pressor agents may increase oxygen consumption and induce myocardial ischemia. The client may also be experiencing pain, because hypotension affects perfusion to all major organs. The nurse will continue to monitor Mr. B.'s vital signs and ECG for any changes and will administer O_2 and morphine for the pain along with nitroglycerin. The nurse will encourage Mr. B. to relax. A sedative is usually ordered if a client is extremely anxious.

CHAPTER 55

Antihypertensive Drugs

MAJOR TOPICS

- Physiology of blood pressure regulation
- Characteristics, risk factors, and causes of hypertension
- Characteristics and types of antihypertensive drugs

QUICK REFERENCE GUIDE TO TEXT

- Objectives, p. 808
- Interactive displays, pp. 808 and 822
- Table 55-1. Antihypertensive drugs, p. 816
- Box 55-1. Mechanisms that regulate blood pressure, p. 809
- Figure 55-1. Actions of ACE inhibitors and angiotensin II receptor antagonists, p. 814
- Nursing process, pp. 815 and 820
- Client teaching guidelines, p. 821
- Principles of therapy, p. 820
- Review and application exercises, p. 829

TERMS AND CONCEPTS

Angiotensin II	Vascular tone
Hypertension	Vasoconstriction
Hypotension	Vasodilation
Peripheral vascular resistance	

DRUG LIST

- Amlodipine (Norvasc)
- Atenolol (Tenormin)
- Captopril (Capoten)
- Clonidine (Catapres)
- Diltiazem (sustained-release) (Cardizem SR, Dilacor XR)
- Doxazosin (Cardura)
- Losartan (Cozaar)
- Metoprolol (Lopressor)
- Verapamil (Calan, Calan SR, Verelan)

■ Teaching Strategies

CLASSROOM

1. Lecture/discussion, using the objectives as an outline. The topic of hypertension and its management warrants 1 or more class periods because of its common occurrence, its potentially serious consequences, the numerous types of drugs used to treat it, and the important role of nurses in drug therapy.

2. Show a transparency of the major groups of antihypertensive drugs (transparency 44), and review the mechanism by which each group lowers blood pressure.

3. With calcium channel blockers, emphasize that only sustained-release forms of diltiazem and nifedipine are approved for treatment of hypertension. In addition, sustained-release forms of these drugs are available in different dosage strengths (diltiazem in 60-, 90-, 120-, 180-, 240-, and 300-mg capsules; nifedipine in 30-, 60-, and 90-mg tablets) and with different abbreviations (eg, Cardizem SR, Cardizem CD, Dilacor XR, Adalat CC, Procardia XL). Emphasize the need for careful comparison of drug orders and available formulations before administration, and emphasize that sustained-release forms should not be crushed, bitten, chewed, or opened (capsules).

4. Show a transparency of the mechanism of action of ACE inhibitors and angiotensin II receptor antagonists (transparency 45).

5. Prepare and show a transparency of ACE inhibitors (eg, captopril as the prototype, others commonly used in local clinical practice agencies).

6. Ask students about their experiences with hypertensive clients or family members.

7. Emphasize the importance of accurate measurement of blood pressure. Ask students whether they have observed errors in technique and, if so, to describe the errors.

8. Ask an adult client with hypertension to speak to the class about personal perceptions of the disease, its treatment, and helpful or nonhelpful behaviors of nurses and other health care providers.

COLLABORATIVE ACTIVITIES FOR SMALL GROUPS

1. Noncompliance with drug therapy is a major problem in the treatment of hypertension. Ask groups to list possible reasons for noncompliance and possible nursing interventions to promote compliance, as many as they can in 5 or 10 minutes. Then list these on a marker board and discuss them as a class (eg, which reasons are most likely, the ease or difficulty of implementing particular nursing interventions).

2. Discuss review and application exercises 9, 10, and 11 (text, p. 829).

3. Discuss the Critical Thinking Case Study (study guide, p. 179).

CLINICAL LABORATORY

1. Have students measure blood pressure for all assigned clients and compare the values with previously recorded values.

2. For clients with hypertension, have students assess for personal characteristics and lifestyle habits that may cause or aggravate hypertension and decrease the effectiveness of antihypertensive drugs.

3. For clients receiving antihypertensive drugs, have students measure blood pressure before and after administering the drugs. This helps in assessing clients' responses to the medications.

4. For clients receiving antihypertensive drugs, identify OTC drugs that can increase or decrease blood pressure.

5. For clients receiving antihypertensive drugs, analyze all prescribed medications for those that may increase or decrease blood pressure.

6. Ask students to identify assigned clients who are receiving a combination of antihypertensive drugs. In postclinical conference, discuss various combinations and clients' responses to the therapy.

7. For assigned clients with a newly prescribed antihypertensive drug, ask students to individualize agency or pharmacy instructions.

8. In preclinical conference, ask students to observe agency staff measuring blood pressure, and evaluate their techniques for accuracy or error. Common errors include using a cuff of the wrong size, applying the cuff too loosely or over clothing; having the arm higher or lower than heart level or not supporting the arm adequately; and reinflating the cuff before it deflates completely.

9. In preclinical or postclinical conference, ask 2 students to demonstrate blood pressure measurement, with some planned errors in technique. Ask other students to evaluate the technique and, when errors are noted, to describe the correct technique.

■ Critical Thinking Case Study

1. Exercise will help M. lose weight and decrease her blood pressure. A reduction in dietary sodium and cessation of smoking would also be important goals.

2. Atenolol (Tenormin), a selective beta blocker, is a commonly used first-line antihypertensive medication. Beta blockers decrease renin levels.

3. I would instruct the client to have her blood pressure checked at least once a week (or daily if required) while her antihypertensive regime is evaluated, or purchase a self-monitoring blood pressure unit and report to her physician by telephone.

4. She should be encouraged to keep track of her weight and her dietary intake. A support group such as Weight Watchers may be beneficial.

5. M. was not well controlled on Inderal. Rather than increase the medication and increase the risk of side effects, the physician changed M.'s medication. In clients with renal disease, ACE inhibitors are effective. Diuretics are often added to combat sodium, potassium, and fluid retention.

CHAPTER 56

Diuretics

MAJOR TOPICS

- Renal physiology
- Conditions for which diuretics are used
- Types of diuretic drugs

QUICK REFERENCE GUIDE TO TEXT

TERMS AND CONCEPTS

Ascites	Hyperglycemia
Diuresis	Hyperkalemia
Edema	Hyperuricemia
Hypokalemia	

DRUG LIST

- Furosemide (Lasix)
- Hydrochlorothiazide (HydroDIURIL)
- Hydrochlorothiazide/triamterene (Dyazide, Maxzide)
- Mannitol (Osmitrol)

■ Teaching Strategies

CLASSROOM

1. Lecture/discussion using the objectives as an outline. Show transparencies of Figures 56-1 and 56-2 (transparencies 46 and 47 to review renal physiology and illustrate sites of action of diuretic drugs.

2. Ask students about their experiences with clients receiving diuretics.

3. Remind students that the generic names of all the thiazide diuretics end in "-thiazide."

4. For clients receiving diuretics, discuss assessing their conditions for therapeutic and adverse drug effects.

5. Review signs and symptoms of fluid volume deficit.

6. Warn students that diuretics are sometimes misused/abused for weight control and discuss the dangers of such use.

COLLABORATIVE ACTIVITIES FOR SMALL GROUPS

1. Prepare a teaching plan for a client being started on diuretic therapy.

2. Discuss selected review and application exercises (text, p. 846).

3. Compare and contrast the use of diuretics in children, in older adults, and in clients with impaired renal or hepatic function.

4. Discuss the Critical Thinking Case Study (study guide, p. 183).

CLINICAL LABORATORY

1. For clients receiving a diuretic, have students assess for signs and symptoms of dehydration.

2. For clients receiving a diuretic, have students check laboratory reports for serum potassium concentration, hematocrit, urine specific gravity, and other indicators of fluid and electrolyte status.

3. Show students a urine sample and ask what conclusions they can draw about the client's hydration status.

4. Have students administer diuretics and observe clients' responses.

■ Critical Thinking Case Study

1. Lasix was ordered to diurese Mr. P., resulting in decreased preload, decreased serum potassium levels, and decreased stress on the heart. Aldactone is a potassium-sparing diuretic that induces fluid loss but retains potassium. Administration of these two drugs cause substantial fluid loss without hypokalemia. Digoxin increases the force of contraction of the heart and the cardiac output.

2. The following assessments should be done: heart rate and rhythm, urinary output, weight, blood pressure, breath sounds, peripheral pulses, skin temperature, digoxin level, potassium level, and creatinine level.

3. Perform a complete head-to-toe assessment. If possible, given your facility, obtain an O_2 saturation measurement. Review all recent laboratory work and chart data. Have a list of Mr. P.'s medications and all the assessment information available when you contact his physician.

CHAPTER 57

Drugs That Affect Blood Coagulation

MAJOR TOPICS

- Physiology of hemostasis and thrombosis
- Platelet activation, adhesion, and aggregation
- Role of atherosclerosis and endothelial cells in thrombosis
- Venous and arterial thrombotic disorders
- Blood clotting factors
- Anticoagulant, antiplatelet, and thrombolytic drugs
- Hemostatic agents

QUICK REFERENCE GUIDE TO TEXT

- Objectives, p. 847
- Interactive displays, pp. 847, 853, and 860
- Table 57-1. Blood coagulation factors, p. 848
- Table 57-2. Anticoagulant, antiplatelet, and thrombolytic agents, p. 852
- Table 57-3. Systemic hemostatic drugs, p. 857
- Box 57-1. Hemostasis and thrombosis, p. 849
- Nursing process, pp. 857 and 859
- Client teaching guidelines, p. 859
- Principles of therapy, p. 860
- Review and application exercises, p. 867

TERMS AND CONCEPTS

Activated partial thromboplastin time (APTT)	Hemostasis
Antiplatelet effects	Prothrombin time (PT)
Coagulation	Thromboembolic
Embolus	Thrombolytic
	Thrombus

DRUG LIST

- Alteplase recombinant (t-PA) (Activase)
- Aminocaproic acid (Amicar)
- Aspirin
- Clopidogrel (Plavix)
- Enoxaparin (Lovenox)
- Heparin
- Protamine sulfate
- Vitamin K
- Warfarin (Coumadin)

■ Teaching Strategies

CLASSROOM

1. Lecture/discussion, using the objectives as an outline. Show transparency 48 to focus students' attention and provide an overview of drugs used to treat thromboembolic disorders.

2. Show a transparency comparing heparin and warfarin (transparency 49).

3. Discuss the nursing care of clients who are receiving heparin and warfarin, including administering the drug, observing responses, and teaching self-administration and monitoring.

4. Identify foods and medications, including OTC products, to be avoided by clients taking warfarin.

5. Review antiplatelet effects of aspirin.

6. Emphasize that most myocardial infarctions are caused by blood clots in the coronary arteries and that thrombolytic agents can limit the extent of

infarction if given within a few hours after onset of chest pain.

COLLABORATIVE ACTIVITIES FOR SMALL GROUPS

1. Have each group discuss 1 or 2 review and application exercises (text, p. 867) and share their findings with the class as a whole.

2. Discuss the use of anticoagulants and antiplatelet drugs for clients with renal or hepatic impairment.

3. Prepare a teaching plan for a client who is beginning warfarin therapy.

4. Discuss the Critical Thinking Case Study (study guide, p. 185).

CLINICAL LABORATORY

1. For clients receiving heparin or warfarin, ask students whether the drug is being given for prophylactic or therapeutic purposes.

2. For clients receiving intravenous heparin, have students list activated partial thromboplastin time (APTT) results and identify therapeutic values.

3. For clients receiving warfarin, have students list prothrombin time (PT) and international normalized ratio (INR) results; identify subtherapeutic, therapeutic, or high values; and state the nursing process implications of each.

4. For clients who experience excessive bleeding while taking an anticoagulant, ask students what they would assess for (ie, specific signs and symptoms) and what interventions they would perform.

5. For a hospitalized client being discharged on Coumadin, have a student do the discharge teaching and share the content, format, and teaching techniques with other students during postconference discussion.

■ Critical Thinking Case Study

1. Stay with the client and remain calm. Elevate the head of the bed. Obtain an O_2 saturation measurement if ordered. Administer O_2. If the client is being monitored, get an ECG strip. Contact the physician.

2. M.'s risk factors include sedentary lifestyle, fractured femur, birth control pills, smoking, and possible peripheral vascular disease secondary to diabetes mellitus.

3. Administer both medications. It takes 2 to 3 days before a therapeutic level of Coumadin is reached. Initially the dose of Coumadin is determined by daily PT levels or INR determinations. With long-term use, the tests are performed monthly.

CHAPTER 58

Drugs for Hyperlipidemia

MAJOR TOPICS

- Role of hyperlipidemia in developing atherosclerosis
- Types of hyperlipoproteinemia
- Types of antilipemic drugs
- Prevention and management of hyperlipidemia

QUICK REFERENCE GUIDE TO TEXT

- Objectives, p. 868
- Interactive displays, pp. 868 and 876
- Table 58-1. NCEP recommendations for treatment of hyperlipidemia, p. 872
- Table 58-2. Antilipemic agents, p. 873
- Box 58-1. Types of lipoproteins, p. 870
- Box 58-2. Types of hyperlipidemia, p. 871
- Nursing process, pp. 874 and 875
- Client teaching guidelines, p. 875
- Principles of therapy, p. 876
- Review and application exercises, p. 880

TERMS AND CONCEPTS

Antilipemic	Hypercholesterolemia
Atherosclerosis	Hyperlipidemia
Blood lipids	Triglycerides
Claudication	Viscosity

DRUG LIST

- Atorvastatin (Lipitor)
- Cholestyramine (Questran)
- Gemfibrozil (Lopid)
- Lovastatin (Mevacor)
- Niacin

■ Teaching Strategies

CLASSROOM

1. Lecture/discussion, using the objectives as an outline. Show a transparency of "statin" drugs (transparency 50) as a commonly used group.

2. Ask students what they already know about cholesterol and atherosclerosis.

COLLABORATIVE ACTIVITIES FOR SMALL GROUPS

1. Prepare a teaching plan for a client starting on a "statin."

2. Discuss the review and application exercises (text, p. 880).

CLINICAL LABORATORY

1. Have students list total, LDL, and HDL cholesterol values for several clients. Then, have them analyze the values in terms of risk of cardiovascular disease, whether changes are needed, and how changes can be made.

2. For clients receiving a cholesterol-lowering drug, have students teach ways to increase effectiveness and decrease adverse drug reactions.

3. Have students discuss their dietary intake and evaluate their risk for developing cardiovascular disease.

DRUGS AFFECTING THE DIGESTIVE SYSTEM

CHAPTER 59

Physiology of the Digestive System

MAJOR TOPICS

- Organs and secretions of the GI tract and accessory organs
- Effects of drugs on the GI tract
- Effects of GI disorders on drug absorption

QUICK REFERENCE GUIDE TO TEXT

- Objectives, p. 883
- Review and application exercises, p. 886

TERMS AND CONCEPTS

Catabolism	Metabolism
Enterogastrone	Peristalsis
Gastrin	

■ Teaching Strategies

CLASSROOM

1. Assign students to review GI physiology independently; provide an opportunity to ask questions.

2. Have students write answers to the review and application exercises (text, p. xxx).

CLINICAL LABORATORY

1. For any group of clients, have students list medical diagnoses and prescribed drugs; then, have students identify those diagnoses and drugs associated with adverse effects on the GI system.

2. Have students review clients' medical records for results of liver function tests and verbalize or write the nursing implications of any abnormal values.

CHAPTER 60

Drugs Used in Peptic Ulcer Disease

MAJOR TOPICS

- Characteristics of peptic ulcer disease
- Role of *Helicobacter pylori* organisms
- Types of drugs used to treat peptic ulcer disease

QUICK REFERENCE GUIDE TO TEXT

- Objectives, p. 887
- Interactive displays, pp. 887, 893, and 894
- Table 60-1. Antacids, p. 890
- Table 60-2. Antiulcer drugs, p. 891
- Box 60-1. Selected upper GI disorders, p. 888
- Nursing process, pp. 894 and 895
- Client teaching guidelines, p. 896
- Principles of therapy, p. 895
- Review and application exercises, p. 902

TERMS AND CONCEPTS

Antacid	Prostaglandin
Autodigestion	Proton pump inhibitors
Cytoprotective	Pyrosis
Gastroesophageal reflux disease	Ulcerogenic
Histamine$_2$ receptor blocking agents	

DRUG LIST

- Aluminum hydroxide/magnesium hydroxide (Mylanta)
- Lansoprazole (Prevacid)
- Ranitidine (Zantac)
- Sucralfate (Carafate)

■ Teaching Strategies

CLASSROOM

1. Identify populations at risk for peptic ulcer disease.
2. Show a transparency of antiulcer drugs (transparency 51).
3. Ask students about their experiences with clients receiving antiulcer drugs.
4. Discuss the pathophysiology of gastroesophageal reflux disease (GERD).
5. Discuss the differences in using histamine$_2$ receptor antagonists for peptic ulcer disease and for heartburn.

COLLABORATIVE ACTIVITIES FOR SMALL GROUPS

1. Prepare a teaching plan for a client being started on a prescription histamine$_2$ receptor antagonist, a proton pump inhibitor, or sucralfate.
2. Discuss the review and application exercises (text, p. 902).
3. Discuss the Critical Thinking Case Study (study guide, p. 195).

CLINICAL LABORATORY

1. For a group of clients, have students identify those at risk for peptic ulcer disease or GERD.
2. Have students administer antiulcer drugs and report the procedure and client responses to the clinical group.
3. For a client with a GI drainage tube, have students assess type, amount, and color of any secretions, evaluate them as normal or abnormal, and state nursing interventions needed, if any.

■ Critical Thinking Case Study

1. Mr. J. is given Tagamet because it is an H_2 antagonist. It decreases both the amount and the acidity (hydrogen ion concentration) of gastric juices. It promotes healing, usually within 6–8 weeks. It is also effective in controlling GI bleeding due to peptic ulcer disease.

2. 10 gtt = 1 ml; therefore, in 100 mL there would be 1000 gtt. 1000 gtt / 20 minutes = 50 gtt/min.

3. The nurse should observe for the following adverse reactions in clients who are using Tagamet: CNS—confusion, dizziness, headache, drowsiness; CV—bradycardia; GI—nausea, diarrhea, constipation, hepatitis; GU—nephritis; DERM—rashes, exfoliative dermatitis, urticaria; ENDO—gynecomastia; HEMAT—agranulocytosis, aplastic anemia, neutropenia, thrombocytopenia, anemia; MS—muscle pain. Drug interactions: there are many.

4. Carafate is a unique drug for short-term treatment of duodenal ulcer. It is a preparation of sulfated sucrose and aluminum hydroxide gel that promotes healing of duodenal ulcers. It combines with ulcer exudates, adheres to the ulcer site, and forms a protective coating that decreases further damage by gastric acid, pepsin, and bile salts. You should assess Mr. J. for constipation and dry mouth.

5. Diet therapy has little role in prevention or treatment of peptic ulcer disease. The client should avoid foods that he finds cause him gastric discomfort. However, the client should be cautioned against using so-called "ulcer diets" or bland diets. These diets usually contain large amounts of milk and milk products. Many people consider milk an "antacid" or buffer of gastric acid; however, it has little effect on the pH of gastric juices, and the protein and calcium in milk products induce hypersecretion of gastric acid. Therefore, a diet regimen that includes milk may actually aggravate peptic ulcer disease. Some suggest that clients should avoid highly spiced foods, gas-forming foods, and caffeine-containing beverages.

6. Instructions that should be given to Mr. J. before discharge are as follows: avoid situations that cause or exacerbate symptoms; observe for GI bleeding and other complications of peptic ulcer disease; maintain normal patterns of bowel movements; incorporate relaxation techniques into your lifestyle; continue with the course of therapy for 4–8 weeks to ensure ulcer healing; if a dose is missed, take it as soon as you remember unless it is almost time for the next dose; do not double doses; cessation of smoking may decrease recurrence of ulcers. Emphasize the importance of routine examinations to monitor progress.

CHAPTER 61

Laxatives and Cathartics

MAJOR TOPICS

- Constipation
- Defecation
- Types and characteristics of laxatives

QUICK REFERENCE GUIDE TO TEXT

- Objectives, p. 904
- Interactive displays, pp. 904, 907, and 909
- Table 61-1. Laxatives and Cathartics, p. 906
- Nursing process, p. 908
- Client teaching guidelines: Laxatives, p. 909
- Principles of therapy, p. 909
- Review and application exercises, p. 912

TERMS AND CONCEPTS

Bowel cleansing   Laxative dependence
Laxative abuse

DRUG LIST

- Bisacodyl (Dulcolax)
- Docusate (Colace)
- Milk of magnesia
- Polyethylene glycol-electrolyte solution (CoLyte)
- Psyllium (Effersyllium, Metamucil)

■ Teaching Strategies

CLASSROOM

1. This content may be familiar to most students, so a few minutes may be sufficient to emphasize the main points.

2. Lecture/discussion, using the objectives as an outline.

COLLABORATIVE ACTIVITIES FOR SMALL GROUPS

1. Discuss possible interventions with a friend who abuses laxatives to control weight.

2. Design a bowel management regimen for a client with cancer who requires large doses of opioid analgesics to control pain.

3. Discuss the review and application exercises (text, p. 912).

4. Discuss the Critical Thinking Case Study (study guide, p. 198).

CLINICAL LABORATORY

1. For a group of clients, ask students to identify clients with risk factors for constipation.

2. Have students assess all assigned clients in relation to bowel elimination. For clients with apparent constipation, have students describe interventions to relieve the condition and to prevent its recurrence.

3. Have students interview clients regarding their use of OTC laxatives (eg, type, frequency of use) and their willingness to use nondrug interventions.

■ Critical Thinking Case Study

1. Increased fluid intake, exercise, and roughage can help constipation.

2. Common causes of constipation include immobility, dehydration, diet, and medications.

3. A laxative or glycerin suppository would be a good place to start. If these are not effective, then a Dulcolax suppository or a Fleet Enema may be necessary. After this problem has been resolved, a stool softener may be helpful.

CHAPTER 62

Antidiarrheals

MAJOR TOPICS

- Characteristics and causes of diarrhea
- Types of antidiarrheal drugs

QUICK REFERENCE GUIDE TO TEXT

- Objectives, p. 914
- Interactive displays, pp. 914, 919, and 922
- Table 62-1. Antidiarrheal drugs, p. 916
- Nursing process, pp. 920 and 921
- Client teaching guidelines: Antidiarrheal medications, p. 921
- Principles of therapy, p. 921
- Review and application exercises, p. 924

TERMS AND CONCEPTS

Infectious diarrhea
Pseudomembranous colitis
Inflammatory bowel diseases

DRUG LIST

- Diphenoxylate/atropine (Lomotil)
- Loperamide (Imodium)

■ Teaching Strategies

CLASSROOM

1. This content may be familiar to most students, so a few minutes may be sufficient to emphasize the main points.

2. Lecture/discussion, using the objectives as an outline.

3. Discuss the review and application exercises (text, p. 924).

CLINICAL LABORATORY

1. For a group of clients, ask students to identify clients with risk factors for diarrhea.

2. Have students assess all assigned clients in relation to bowel elimination. For clients who have diarrhea, have students observe characteristics (eg, frequency, amount, consistency, whether mucus, blood, or other abnormal components are present) when possible.

3. Have students assess fluid and electrolyte balance of clients with diarrhea, including laboratory reports if available.

■ Critical Thinking Case Study

1. Your tumor is causing the diarrhea. You can eat foods that are constipating, such as tea, toast, white rice, and bananas. We can try to control it with medication, but we cannot eliminate it. You need to use meticulous skin care.

2. Metamucil when administered with small amounts of fluids is constipating.

3. Assess for dehydration, weight loss, and skin breakdown.

4. Morphine will help control his abdominal pain as well as his diarrhea. This is an appropriate dose for a terminally ill client, and it will probably be adjusted upward.

CHAPTER 63

● **Antiemetics**

MAJOR TOPICS

- Characteristics and causes of nausea and vomiting
- Types of antiemetic drugs

QUICK REFERENCE GUIDE TO TEXT

TERMS AND CONCEPTS

Chemoreceptor trigger zone
Emetogenic
Prokinetic

DRUG LIST

- Metoclopramide (Reglan)
- Ondansetron (Zofran)
- Promethazine (Phenergan)

■ Teaching Strategies

CLASSROOM

1. Lecture/discussion, using the objectives as an outline. Ondansetron and related drugs are usually considered the most effective drugs to manage postoperative and chemotherapy-associated nausea and vomiting (transparency 52).

2. Emphasize the importance of nursing decision-making in administering antiemetic drugs before emetogenic events and PRN.

3. Emphasize that most antiemetic agents cause sedation and that interventions to protect the client may be needed.

4. Discuss the importance of managing nausea and vomiting for clients undergoing emetogenic cancer chemotherapy. This is often a considerable source of anxiety for clients and should be discussed with them before they start chemotherapy.

5. Discuss the review and application exercises (text, p. 935).

CLINICAL LABORATORY

1. For a group of clients, ask students to identify clients with risk factors for nausea and vomiting and to provide interventions to prevent their occurrence.

2. For clients who have nausea, have students administer prescribed antiemetic drugs and observe clients' responses.

3. For clients who vomit, have students observe and record characteristics (eg, frequency, amount, and whether undigested food, blood, or other abnormal components are present) when possible.

4. For clients with extensive vomiting, have students evaluate their fluid and electrolyte status, including laboratory reports when available.

■ Critical Thinking Case Study

1. Ativan does not stop nausea, but it decreases the client's memory of nausea. Thus it helps eliminate anticipatory nausea before a treatment.

2. Small, frequent, high-carbohydrate meals may be helpful. Administration of antiemetics before a chemotherapy treatment is also helpful.

3. Compazine is a phenothiazine that can be administered intramuscularly or rectally. This drug, a CNS depressant, is considered safe for treatment of nausea and vomiting associated with chemotherapy, but it can cause drowsiness.

DRUGS USED IN SPECIAL CONDITIONS

CHAPTER 64

Drugs Used in Oncologic Disorders

MAJOR TOPICS

- Characteristics of normal and malignant cells
- Causes and types of cancer
- Types of anticancer drugs
- Cell cycle effects of anticancer drugs
- Adverse effects of anticancer drugs

QUICK REFERENCE GUIDE TO TEXT

TERMS AND CONCEPTS

Alopecia	Metastasis
Anaplastic	Mucositis
Cell cycle	Nephropathy
Cell differentiation	Neuropathy
Cytotoxic	Neutropenia
Extravasation	Oncogenes and antioncogenes
Leukopenia	Stomatitis
Malignant	Thrombocytopenia

DRUG LIST

- Cisplatin (Platinol)
- Cyclophosphamide (Cytoxan)
- Doxorubicin (Adriamycin)
- Etoposide (VePesid)
- Fluorouracil (Adrucil)
- Methotrexate (Amethopterin)
- Tamoxifen (Nolvadex)
- Vincristine (Oncovin)

■ Teaching Strategies

CLASSROOM

1. If the pathophysiology of cancer and/or nursing care of clients with cancer has been extensively covered in a pathophysiology or medical-surgical nursing class, the instructor can concentrate on anticancer drugs. If this is not the case, discussion of causes, characteristics, and treatment modalities is probably needed, to aid understanding of drug effects. Show transparency 53.

2. Emphasize that cytotoxic antineoplastic chemotherapy is best ordered by physicians, prepared by pharmacists, and administered by nurses who specialize in oncology. Chemotherapy is potential toxic and has stringent requirements for preparation, administration, and client monitoring.

3. Prepare and show a transparency of major groups of anticancer drugs; show transparency 54 to illustrate cell cycle effects.

4. Emphasize individual drugs or groups of drugs that students are likely to encounter in clinical practice.

5. Ask an oncology nurse to speak to the class about the knowledge, skills, and agency requirements for administering anticancer drugs.

6. Ask students to obtain a journal article from an authoritative source (print or Internet) about some aspect of cancer chemotherapy and write a summary to be turned in.

7. Ask a hospice nurse to speak to the class about the hospice philosophy and often-needed nursing interventions for terminally ill clients and their families.

COLLABORATIVE ACTIVITIES FOR SMALL GROUPS

1. Discuss and write answers to the review and application exercises (text, p. 966).

2. Discuss the Critical Thinking Case Study (study guide, p. 208).

CLINICAL LABORATORY

1. For clients receiving anticancer chemotherapy, have students list drugs, look up unfamiliar drugs in a reference book, and analyze the information to determine potential adverse drug effects. Then, observe and interview clients and review laboratory reports for values indicating adverse drug effects.

2. For clients newly prescribed outpatient intravenous anticancer drug therapy, teach what to expect in terms of where, when, and by whom medications will be given. Also, teach about possible adverse drug effects and how they can be prevented or managed.

3. For outpatients receiving oral anticancer drugs, have students interview clients regarding their attitude toward the medication regimen, any problems associated with the drug therapy, degree of compliance with the prescribed therapy, and whether health care providers are seen as supportive.

4. Assign students to spend a day with a nurse in a clinic or physician's office who administers antineoplastic chemotherapy. Have students write a short description of their observations and feelings about the experience.

■ Critical Thinking Case Study

1. It is common to use several drugs to attack a cancer at various places in the cell cycle. Fluorouracil causes hair loss and stomatitis. Mrs. J. should make arrangements for a wig before she loses her hair. Bone marrow depression commonly occurs, so laboratory values need to be monitored. An adequate fluid intake will help minimize the hemorrhagic cystitis that results from Cytoxan administration.

2. Allow her to express her feelings about her body image change. Ask her if she would like to speak with a cancer survivor. Stomatitis can be treated with room-temperature foods, Xylocaine Viscous, and Carafate.

3. Cytoxan can cause hemorrhagic cystitis. Contact her physician and force fluids.

4. These symptoms can be indicative of heart failure. The physician should be contacted immediately.

CHAPTER 65

Drugs Used in Ophthalmic Conditions

MAJOR TOPICS

- Structures of the eye
- Ophthalmic disorders
- Types of ophthalmic drugs

QUICK REFERENCE GUIDE TO TEXT

TERMS AND CONCEPTS

Conjunctiva	Mydriasis
Glaucoma	Refraction
Miosis	Tonometry

DRUG LIST

- Glycerin (Osmoglyn)
- Timolol (Timoptic)
- Tropicamide (Mydriacyl)

■ Teaching Strategies

CLASSROOM

1. Lecture/discussion, using the objectives as an outline.

2. Discuss unique features of administering and observing the effects of ophthalmic medications.

3. Discuss drug therapy for a client with glaucoma, cataract surgery, or eye infection and the subsequent nursing process implications.

COLLABORATIVE ACTIVITIES FOR SMALL GROUPS

1. Prepare a teaching plan for a client being started on eye drops.

2. Discuss review and application exercises 3, 4, and 5 (text, p. 982).

CLINICAL LABORATORY

1. For clients receiving eye medications, have students verbalize the correct techniques, administer the drugs, and observe for systemic effects (eg, bradycardia with beta blockers).

2. Have students teach clients self-administration of eye drops and ointments.

3. Have students participate in vision screening programs in health fairs or schools.

■ Critical Thinking Case Study

1. Pilocarpine is a cholinergic agent that increases the outflow of aqueous humor. Timoptic is a beta-

adrenergic blocker that decreases the production of aqueous humor and thereby decreases intraocular pressure.

2. It is important that you take the drops at the prescribed times. Failure to take the medication can jeopardize your vision. Your night vision will be affected; it is not advisable to drive after dark. You should avoid any medication that will increase your intraocular pressure. Make sure that you make all

of your health care providers aware that you have glaucoma.

3. You will need to use the medication the rest of your life.

4. Glaucoma is hereditary, but if it is caught early damage can be prevented. Your children should be screened yearly.

CHAPTER 66

Drugs Used in Dermatologic Conditions

MAJOR TOPICS

- Functions of skin and mucous membranes
- Skin disorders
- Types of dermatologic drugs

QUICK REFERENCE GUIDE TO TEXT

- Objectives, p. 983
- Interactive displays, pp. 983, 993, and 997
- Table 66-1. Topical antimicrobial agents, p. 987
- Table 66-2. Topical corticosteroids, p. 989
- Table 66-3. Miscellaneous dermatologic agents, p. 992
- Nursing process, pp. 988–991
- Client teaching guidelines, p. 992
- Principles of therapy, p. 993
- Review and application exercises, p. 998

TERMS AND CONCEPTS

Acne	Psoriasis
Candidiasis	Rosacea
Dermatitis	Tinea pedis
Dermatophytosis	Urticaria
Pruritus	

DRUG LIST

- Acyclovir (Zovirax)
- Benzoyl peroxide (Oxy 5, Panoxyl)
- Hydrocortisone (Cortril, others)
- Metronidazole (MetroLotion)
- Povidone-iodine (Betadine)

■ Teaching Strategies

CLASSROOM

1. Lecture/discussion, using the objectives as an outline.

2. Discuss unique features of administering dermatologic medications.

3. Discuss drug therapy for a client with a skin disorder, such as acne or dermatitis, and the associated nursing process implications.

COLLABORATIVE ACTIVITIES FOR SMALL GROUPS

1. Prepare a teaching plan for a client who is to use a topical corticosteroid with an occlusive dressing at home.

2. Discuss review and application exercises 3, 4, 6, and 7 (text, pp. 998–999).

3. Discuss the Critical Thinking Case Study (study guide, p. 215).

CLINICAL LABORATORY

1. Have students assess clients (especially those who are elderly or debilitated or whose activities are restricted) for skin disorders such as pressure ulcers.

2. For clients receiving dermatologic medications, have students verbalize the correct techniques, administer the drugs, and observe responses.

3. Have students teach clients how to cleanse the skin and apply dermatologic drugs.

4. Have students participate in teaching adolescent groups the facts and myths associated with acne.

5. Have students teach caregivers of elderly or debilitated clients the importance and techniques of preventing pressure ulcers.

■ Critical Thinking Case Study

1. Wash your face gently and apply the medication topically once a day. It is an irritant, so your face will appear red.

2. Emotional stress and use of birth control pills can aggravate acne. Talk to your physician about changing your medication.

3. Instruct her to stop using the medication and to apply clean, cold compresses to her face until it has healed. Ask her how she has been using the medication. Ask her whether she has any symptoms of hypervitaminosis A: nausea, vomiting, headache, blurred vision, eye irritation, or muscle skeletal pain.

CHAPTER 67

Drug Use During Pregnancy and Lactation

MAJOR TOPICS

- Maternal-placental-fetal circulation
- Maternal changes of pregnancy
- Drug effects during pregnancy
- Fetal therapeutics
- Management of pregnancy-induced symptoms
- Management of chronic diseases during pregnancy
- Neonatal therapeutics
- Drugs used during labor, delivery, and lactation

QUICK REFERENCE GUIDE TO TEXT

- Objectives, p. 1000
- Interactive displays, pp. 1000 and 1013
- Table 67-1. Pregnancy: Physiologic and pharmacokinetic changes, p. 1001
- Box 67-1. FDA drug categories regarding pregnancy, p. 1002
- Table 67-2. Drug effects in pregnancy, p. 1003
- Table 67-3. Abortifacients, tocolytics, and oxytocics, p. 1010
- Table 67-4. Drug effects in lactation, p. 1014
- Figure 67-1. Fetal development, p. 1002
- Nursing process, pp. 1012 and 1013
- Client teaching guidelines, p. 1013
- Principles of therapy, p. 1013
- Review and application exercises, p. 1019

TERMS AND CONCEPTS

Abortifacient	Prostaglandins
Oxytocic	Tocolytic

DRUG LIST

- Carboprost (Hemabate)
- Oxytocin (Pitocin)
- Ritodrine (Yutopar)
- Terbutaline (Brethine)

■ Teaching Strategies

CLASSROOM

1. If there is a separate pharmacology course, review the course syllabus and talk with the instructor of obstetric nursing regarding drug-related content to promote needed coverage and avoid unnecessary repetition. Show transparency 55 to review fetal development.

2. Discuss the hazards of taking any drugs, smoking cigarettes, or drinking alcohol during pregnancy or if sexually active and not using effective contraception.

3. Emphasize the nursing role in teaching pregnant women nondrug-related interventions to relieve pregnancy-induced symptoms.

COLLABORATIVE ACTIVITIES FOR SMALL GROUPS

1. Discuss the review and application exercises (text, p. 1019).

2. Discuss the Critical Thinking Case Study (study guide, p. 218).

3. Share opinions and attitudes about abortion and the nurse's role in caring for clients undergoing abortion; then, discuss this subject as a class.

CLINICAL LABORATORY

1. Have students teach adolescent and adult women of reproductive potential about the desirability of avoiding drugs, including OTC preparations, when there is any chance of becoming pregnant.

2. Have students assist with prenatal assessment, monitoring, and teaching in an obstetric clinic or physician's office.

3. For a group of prenatal clients, have students list the drugs being taken and evaluate their teratogenic potential.

4. Assign students to prepare a nursing care plan or write a short paper about drug therapy for pregnant clients with chronic diseases such as asthma, diabetes mellitus, epilepsy, or hypertension.

■ Critical Thinking Case Study

1. The suppository will "ripen" your cervix, causing it to dilate more easily, and the oxytocin will induce contractions.

2. Evaluate her pain. Help her to use her Lamaze breathing. Discuss with her the implications for labor if she receives pain medication.

3. Stop the administration of the pain medication and immediately check her vital signs. If her blood pressure has dropped, place her on her side and administer O_2. Check the fetal heart rate, and then contact the physician.

■ Web Sites for Drug and Other Health-Related Information

- Agency for Healthcare Research and Quality (AHRQ), formerly Agency for Health Care Policy and Research
  http://www.ahcpr.gov
- American Cancer Society
  http://www.cancer.org
- American College of Cardiology
  http://www.acc.org
- American Diabetes Association
  http://www.diabetes.org
- Arthritis Foundation
  http://www.arthritis.org
- Centers for Disease Prevention and Control
  http://www.cdc.gov
- Cystic Fibrosis Foundation
  http://www.cff.org
- CBS Healthwatch
  http://cbshealthwatch.medscape.com
- Food and Drug Administration (Department of Health and Human Services)
  http://www.fda.gov
- Healthfinder (Department of Health and Human Services, Office of Disease Prevention and Health Promotion)
  http://www.healthfinder.gov

- HIV/AIDS Treatment Information Service
  http://www.hivatis.org
- InteliHealth
  http://www.intelihealth.com
- Leukemia Society of American
  http://www.leukemia.org
- Mayday Pain Resource Center
  http://mayday.coh.org
- Mayo Clinic Health Oasis (includes a prescription-drug index)
  http://www.mayohealth.org
- MedlinePlus (National Library of Medicine)
  http://www.nlm.nih.gov/medlineplus
- Medscape
  http://www.medscape.com
- National Cancer Institute
  http://www.nci.nih.gov
- National Institutes of Health
  http://www.nih.gov/health
- National Library of Medicine
  http://www.nlm.nih.gov
- National Stroke Association
  http://www.stroke.org
- OncoLink (University of Pennsylvania Cancer Center)
  http://www.oncolink.upenn.edu
- Pharmaceutical Information Network
  http://www.pharminfo.com

Testbank

CHAPTER 1

1. The following drug is derived from a plant:
   - *a. morphine
   - b. iron
   - c. insulin
   - d. penicillin

2. A naturally occurring substance that has been chemically modified is a
   - a. synthetic drug
   - *b. semisynthetic drug
   - c. manipulated drug
   - d. natural drug

3. Each hybrid molecule produces a genetically identical molecule called a
   - a. protein product
   - b. gene
   - *c. clone
   - d. demyelinated cell

4. Morphine is classified as all of the following except
   - a. CNS depressant
   - b. opioid analgesic
   - c. opiate
   - *d. anti-inflammatory agent

5. The drug name patented by the manufacturer is the
   - *a. trade name
   - b. chemical name
   - c. official name
   - d. generic name

6. A reference book that provides information from the drug manufacturers' inserts is the
   - a. American Formulary Service
   - b. Drug Facts and Comparisons
   - *c. Physicians' Desk Reference
   - d. United States Pharmacopeia

7. The first federal law that regulated drug products was the
   - a. Controlled Substance Act
   - b. Food, Drug and Cosmetic Act
   - c. Harrison Narcotic Act
   - *d. Pure Food and Drug Act

8. The following organization regulates vaccines:
   - a. Food and Drug Administration (FDA)
   - *b. Public Health Service
   - c. Federal Trade Commission
   - d. Occupational Safety and Health Administration (OSHA)

9. In phase I of clinical drug trials, potential uses and effects are determined by
   - *a. giving doses to healthy volunteers
   - b. giving doses to persons with the disease
   - c. double blind studies
   - d. crossover studies

10. This cellular structure stores hormones and other substances:
    - a. lysosomes
    - b. endoplasmic reticulum
    - c. mitochondria
    - *d Golgi complex

CHAPTER 2

1. Passive diffusion involves

    *a. the movement of a drug from an area of higher concentration to an area of lower concentration

    b. the drug combining with an enzyme or protein

    c. the movement of a drug from an area of lower concentration to an area of higher concentration

    d. dissolving the lipid layer of the cell membrane so drugs can pass through

2. The process that occurs between the time a drug enters the body and the time it enters the bloodstream is referred to as

    *a. absorption

    b. distribution

    c. metabolism

    d. excretion

3. Drugs formulated to be absorbed through the skin include

    a. amoxicillin, tetracycline, penicillin

    b. insulin, heparin, morphine

    *c. clonidine, fentanyl, estrogen

    d. digoxin, lidocaine, propranolol

4. Distribution of drugs may be altered by

    a. impaired kidney function

    b. accelerated drug metabolism

    c. increased adrenal function

    *d. decreased protein binding

5. Excretion may be increased when

    a. the liver is unable to metabolize lipid soluble drugs

    *b. protein binding is impaired

    c. the client is acidotic

    d. extracellular fluid volume is increased

6. Two medications taken concomitantly with similar effects produce an effect that is the sum of the effects of both medications. This interaction is called

    *a. additive

    b. antagonistic

    c. cumulative

    d. synergistic

7. The blood–brain barrier

    a. allows only IV medications to penetrate into the brain tissues

    b. is highly resistant to water, oxygen, and carbon dioxide

    *c. does not allow many medications to penetrate the brain for therapeutic effect

    d. has no significant implication because the molecules of all medications are so small that they can penetrate the barrier

CHAPTER 3

1. One reason that clients have adverse reactions to medications is because

    a. physicians are not knowledgeable about disease processes in relation to drug therapy

    *b. they may take drugs from several physicians and fail to inform one physician about drugs prescribed by another

    c. nurses have inadequate knowledge about medications and fail to read labels sufficiently

    d. pharmacists dispense incorrect medications and mislabel containers

2. A major disadvantage to using the oral route for drug administration is

    *a. it has a slower rate of action

    b. oral medications have an unpleasant taste

    c. tolerance occurs more frequently

    d. the dose must be doubled

3. The physician orders 2000 U of heparin SC. Heparin comes in 5000 U/mL. How much will you administer?

    a. 0.2 mL

    b. 0.3 mL

    *c. 0.4 mL

    d. 0.5 mL

4. The physician orders 60 mEq to be added to the IV. The container reads 10 mEq/5 mL. How many mL will you administer?

    a. 10 mL

    b. 20 mL

    *c. 30 mL

    d. 40 mL

5. The following gauge needle is commonly used for an IM injection:
   a. 16 gauge
   b. 18 gauge
   *c. 22 gauge
   d. 25 gauge

6. Specify the order of absorption from most rapid to least rapid.
   a. PO, SC, IM, IV
   b. IV, SC, IM, PO
   c. SC, IV, IM, PO
   *d. IV, IM, SC, PO

7. If a medication is ordered to be given intrathecally, it will be administered into the
   a. artery
   b. joint
   *c. cerebrospinal fluid
   d. layers of the skin

8. If a medication is ordered to be administered buccally, you will insert it in the
   a. eye
   b. vagina
   *c. cheek
   d. nose

9. The amount of medication administered intramuscularly should not exceed
   a. 1.5 mL
   b. 2.5 mL
   *c. 3 mL
   d. 5 mL

10. When pouring liquid medication you should
   *a. hold the medication cup at eye level
   b. place the medication cup on the countertop
   c. read the medication at the highest point of the meniscus
   d. pour from the side of the bottle with the label

11. A vaginal suppository is ordered. You will
   a. insert it with its cover
   *b. retrieve it from the refrigerator or drawer
   c. mix it with lubricant before insertion
   d. expect it to be expelled within 10 minutes

12. Tetracycline is ordered q.i.d. for a 3 year old. The best schedule to follow is
   *a. 7 a.m., 11 a.m., 3 p.m., 7 p.m.
   b. 6 a.m., 12 p.m., 6 p.m., 12 a.m.
   c. 8 a.m., 1 p.m., 8 p.m., 1 a.m.
   d. 7 a.m., 2 p.m., 7 p.m., 2 a.m.

13. The physician writes an order: Garamycin gtts 1 in OD. You will administer the drug in the client's
   a. left ear
   b. right ear
   c. left eye
   *d. right eye

14. When administering a narcotic intramuscularly, you should
   a. inject the medication rapidly
   b. insert the needle very slowly
   *c. explain to the client what he or she will feel
   d. inject the medication into a tightened muscle

15. The following route of administration has the fastest rate of absorption:
   a. PO
   b. SC
   c. IM
   *d. inhalation

16. In a toddler, the most important factor when administering medication is the
   a. sex of the child
   b. age of the child
   *c. weight of the child
   d. development of the child

17. A medication given by injection within the subdural space and into the cerebrospinal fluid is administered via the
   a. intraspinal route
   b. intracutaneous route
   c. intra-articular route
   *d. intrathecal route

CHAPTER 4

1. A physical assessment contains
   a. subjective data
   b. objective data
   *c. subjective and objective data
   d. indirect data

2. The following is an example of an expected outcome or goal:
   a. client states she is nauseated, pulse 100, respirations 20
   b. client will increase her level of activity
   c. client at high risk for injury
   *d. client will eat 2000 calories/day by 12/18/00

3. A prototype drug is
   a. a drug that has all of the therapeutic and adverse effects of the classification
   b. the newest drug within a classification
   *c. a drug within a classification that has many common characteristics of the other drugs within the classification
   d. a drug that was originally introduced for one purpose and is now used for a variety of purposes

4. Assessing a client's cultural beliefs and practices will help the nurse to
   a. understand the practices of everyone within that cultural group
   b. determine the beliefs that do not fit with scientific method
   *c. provide appropriate information and care that does not conflict with cultural beliefs
   d. learn how to treat people of that culture

5. Before drug therapy is started, the client should be assessed for all of the following except
   *a. sex and ethnic background
   b. age and weight
   c. health status and pathological conditions
   d. ability to perform activities of daily living

6. Baseline data commonly obtained prior to initiating most drug therapy include
   a. bone marrow function studies
   *b. liver and kidney function studies
   c. blood clotting tests
   d. cardiac enzymes

7. The following is most appropriate when administering medication to children:
   a. if a child is resistant, tell the child that the medication is candy
   b. measurement by teaspoons is as accurate as milliliters
   c. if a drug is not supplied in a liquid form, you can crush it and place it in honey
   *d. allow them to choose a favorite drink to take after the medication

8. The following best describes drug efficacy/toxicity in pediatric clients:
   a. drug requirement for infants has been extensively studied
   *b. drug dosage is altered by disease state and weight in children
   c. children always need smaller doses of medication than adults
   d. infants and children are always at greater risk for drug toxicity with any medication

9. The following is a normal physiologic change associated with aging:
   *a. lean body mass decreases
   b. subcutaneous tissue increases
   c. total body water increases
   d. muscle mass increases

10. Fat-soluble drugs in the elderly
    a. are absorbed at a slower rate
    b. are released more quickly into the circulation
    c. are distributed to a smaller portion of the tissue
    *d. have an increased duration of action

CHAPTER 5

1. Mr. C., who suffered a head injury this morning, is having difficulty breathing. This is a result of swelling around his
   a. thalamus
   b. cerebrum
   c. pituitary
   *d. medulla oblongata

2. When administering morphine, the nurse must assess
   a. peripheral pulses
   b. heart sounds
   c. bowel sounds
   *d. respiratory rate

3. Mr. J., who is admitted for a myocardial infarction, is started on nitroglycerin. His blood pressure drops. This is due to
   a. stimulation of the hypothalamus
   b. pain associated with the infarction
   *c. vasodilation
   d. central nervous system depression

4. The following is a neurotransmitter:
   a. calcium ion
   b. cholinesterase
   *c. acetylcholine
   d. monamine oxidase

5. Hypoxia is due to:
   a. increased synaptic transmission
   *b. interruption of the blood supply
   c. altered neurotransmitter synthesis
   d. neurotransmitter degradation

6. The following are receptors embedded in the cell membranes of neurons:
   *a. proteins
   b. hormones
   c. enzymes
   d. ions

7. Synaptic transmission is increased as a result of
   a. hypokalemia
   b. acidosis
   c. hypocalcemia
   *d. alkalosis

8. This neurotransmitter stimulates the brain to increase activity:
   a. dopamine
   b. acetylcholine
   c. gamma-aminobutyric acid
   *d. norepinephrine

9. A decrease in the following neurotransmitter substance is associated with Parkinson's disease:
   a. acetylcholine
   *b. dopamine
   c. glutamate
   d. serotonin

10. The thalamus
    *a. relays motor impulses from the cortex to the spinal cord
    b. is responsible for voluntary movement
    c. continually adjusts body temperature, blood pressure, and heart rate
    d. helps maintain red blood cell production

11. ADH secretion increases
    a. the osmolarity of the extracellular fluid
    *b. fluid retention
    c. urinary output
    d. the pH of body fluids

12. The following portion of the brain receives impulses from the body, evaluates the impulses, and decides which impulses to transmit to the cerebral cortex:
    *a. reticular activating system
    b. limbic system
    c. pons
    d. medulla oblongata

13. A thiamine deficiency can cause
    *a. reduced glucose use
    b. mental confusion and dizziness
    c. involuntary reflexes
    d. hyperactivity, nervousness, and insomnia

14. When administering CNS depressants, you should assess
    a. peripheral pulses
    b. heart sounds
    c. bowel sounds
    *d. respiratory rate

CHAPTER 6

1. The physician orders 5 mg of morphine (Roxanol) q2h. Roxanol contains 10 mg/mL. How many drops will you administer?
   a. 2 gtts
   b. 4 gtts
   c. 6 gtts
   *d. 8 gtts

2. Mrs. G., who has a PCA pump, states, "I'm afraid to use this device. I'm worried that I will give myself too much medication." Identify the best response:
   a. "The doctor would never order a PCA pump for you if he thought that could happen."
   b. "If you follow the directions that you have been given, that will not happen."
   c. "The PCA device always provides the correct amount, never too much, never too little."
   *d. "The device is preset, therefore you can only receive a specific amount every few minutes."

3. Your client has been taking morphine q2h for chronic pain associated with cancer. It is important to assess him or her for
   a. diarrhea
   *b. respiratory depression
   c. cough
   d. urinary frequency

4. Tylenol #3 consists of acetaminophen (Tylenol) and
   *a. codeine
   b. Phenergan
   c. Advil
   d. Talwin

5. The following drug is used to reverse the effects of opioids:
   *a. naloxone hydrochloride (Narcan)
   b. butorphanol tartrate (Stadol)
   c. buprenorphine (Buprenex)
   d. nalbuphine hydrochloride (Nubain)

6. Long-term administration of opioids will result in
   a. tachycardia
   b. decreased pain perception
   c. irritable bowel syndrome
   *d. tolerance

7. Administration of opioids can cause
   a. ataxia
   b. blurred vision
   *c. hypotension
   d. dysrhythmias

8. Opiates should not be administered to clients with head injuries because they decrease
   *a. pupillary response
   b. urinary output
   c. core body temperature
   d. peripheral vasodilation

9. A common adverse response to the administration of intravenous morphine is
   a. bronchial constriction
   b. hypoxia
   *c. bradypnea
   d. stasis of secretions

10. The following analgesic should be administered to the client who has had a craniotomy:
    *a. acetaminophen with codeine (Tylenol with codeine)
    b. propoxyphene hydrochloride (Darvon)
    c. levorphanol tartrate (Levo-Dromoran)
    d. morphine sulfate (Roxanol)

11. A client with terminal cancer has been receiving morphine sulfate 5 mg IV q4h for the past 3 weeks. She states that the pain is not relieved. You recognize that the reason for this is the client
    a. has developed a dependency on the morphine
    b. is seeking attention
    c. resents the fact that the nurse is healthy
    *d. has developed tolerance to the morphine

12. For which of the following clients would you question the physician's order of IV morphine?
    a. a 78-year-old client with rheumatoid arthritis
    b. a 32-year-old, 2 days postoperative mastectomy client
    c. an 8-year-old burn client
    *d. a 17-year-old client with a head injury

13. The physician orders meperidine (Demerol) 100 mg IM q4h prn, 2 days post injury, for a 30-year-old male client with a fractured leg. You should:
    *a. give the medication as ordered
    b. hold the medication and notify the physician that the dose is too large
    c. hold the medication and notify the physician that the dose is too small
    d. give half the dose now to see what effect it has

14. Your client will receive fentanyl via patch. For management of pain control using this method, the nurse is aware that fentanyl
    *a. lasts 3 days
    b. provides a short duration of relief
    c. has no adverse effects
    d. requires that the respiratory rate be monitored every 4 hours

15. A common side effect of pain therapy with morphine is
    a. paresthesia in lower extremities
    b. occipital headache
    c. increased intracranial pressure
    *d. drowsiness

16. When you question a client with chronic pain about current medications, he states, "I am taking oxycodone/aspirin (Percodan), which used to help, but now the effect lasts for a short time." This probably indicates
    a. addiction
    b. hepatic insufficiency
    c. psychological dependence
    *d. tolerance

17. When administering pain medication to a client, all of the following are appropriate except:
    a. maintain a positive outlook in anticipation of pain relief
    b. encourage the patient to relax and allow the drug to work
    *c. wait until the client shows signs of pain before administering the drug
    d. take advantage of the placebo effect of the drug.

18. If a client has difficulty urinating postoperatively, the following drug may be administered:
    a. droperidol
    *b. neostigmine
    c. levorphanol
    d. naloxone

CHAPTER 7

1. Aspirin works by
    *a. blocking transmission of pain impulse
    b. increasing adrenal function
    c. suppressing the function of the hypothalamus
    d. increasing WBC production

2. Fever can be caused by
    a. sweating
    b. vasodilatation
    *c. dehydration
    d. fluid overload

3. A disorder resulting from elevated uric acid levels is
    a. renal failure
    *b. gout
    c. migraine headaches
    d. diarrhea

4. Migraine headaches result in
    a. vasoconstriction
    b. decreased sensitivity to light and sound
    *c. release of inflammatory mediators
    d. blocked nerve impulses

5. Acetaminophen (Tylenol) is available in all of the following forms except
    a. tablet
    b. liquid
    c. suppository
    *d. patch

6. The following NSAID is available by prescription only:
    a. ibuprofen (Motrin)
    b. ketoprofen (Orudis)
    c. naproxen (Naprosyn)
    *d. flurbiprofen (Ansaid)

7. A potentially serious side effect that a person using indomethacin (Indocin) should be aware of is

    a. agranulocytosis

    *b. bone marrow depression

    c. elevated serum potassium levels

    d. dysrhythmias

8. The only NSAID that can be administered intramuscularly is

    a. etodolac (Lodine)

    b. nabumetone (Relafen)

    c. sulindac (Clinoril)

    *d. ketorolac (Toradol)

9. The following medication treats gout by increasing urinary excretion of uric acid:

    a. allopurinol (Zyloprim)

    *b. probenecid (Benemid)

    c. colchicine

    d. salicylic acid (ASA)

10. Your client has diabetes mellitus, angina, peptic ulcer disease, and asthma. For which one of these problems would you alert the physician before commencing treatment for moderate to severe migraine headaches?

    a. angina

    b. asthma

    *c. peptic ulcer disease

    d. diabetes mellitus

11. Caffeine is mixed with ergotamine in the antimigraine preparation Cafergot because it

    a. decreases blood pressure

    b. promotes relaxation

    c. increases urinary output

    *d. increases vasoconstriction

12. Mr. J, who has sustained a recent musculoskeletal injury, has taken an NSAID; in addition to this, what would you recommend to help control his pain?

    a. relaxation techniques

    *b. application of cold

    c. passive ROM

    d. moist heat

13. A common daily antiplatelet dose of aspirin is

    *a. 81 mg

    b. 180 mg

    c. 360 mg

    d. 600 mg

14. Manifestations of salicylism or salicylate intoxication include

    *a. tinnitus and decreased hearing

    b. hypoventilation and bradycardia

    c. dyspepsia and diarrhea

    d. uncontrolled bleeding from the gums and rectum

15. Treatment for severe salicylate overdose includes

    a. insertion of an NG tube and administration of large quantities of antacids

    b. hyperventilation until the client's pH comes within the appropriate range

    *c. IV sodium bicarbonate

    d. IV loop diuretics

16. A major drawback to acetaminophen is potential

    a. kidney damage

    b. pancreas damage

    c. lung damage

    *d. liver damage

17. The antidote for acetaminophen (Tylenol) poisoning is

    *a. acetylcysteine (Mucomyst)

    b. allopurinol (Zyloprim)

    c. ascorbic acid (Vitamin C)

    d. Amphojel

18. Ingestion of large quantities of NSAIDs over extended periods of time can cause renal impairment. Therefore, the following lab test(s) should be assessed within 2 weeks after initiating therapy:

    a. renin and aldosterone levels

    b. 24-hour urine for microalbumin

    *c. blood urea nitrogen and serum creatinine

    d. LDH and SGOT

19. Disease-modifying antirheumatic drugs have anti-inflammatory and immunosuppressive properties and
    a. decrease the client's sedimentation rate
    b. improve joint deformity
    *c. slow tissue damage
    d. eliminate pain

20. Before surgery, aspirin should be avoided for
    a. 1–2 days
    b. 3–5 days
    *c. 7–10 days
    d. 1 month

21. Aspirin is not recommended for use in children because of its association with
    a. megaloblastic anemia
    b. gastrointestinal bleeding
    *c. Reye's syndrome
    d. growth retardation

CHAPTER 8

1. One of the problems associated with barbiturate use is
    a. impairment of long-term memory
    *b. tolerance and dependence
    c. increase in REM sleep
    d. increased excretion of drugs

2. Most benzodiazepines lose their hypnotic effectiveness with daily use in approximately
    a. 2 weeks
    *b. 1 month
    c. 6 months
    d. 1 year

3. Compared to barbiturates, benzodiazepines do not
    a. produce physiologic dependence or withdrawal symptoms
    *b. suppress REM sleep
    c. cause sedation
    d. precipitate respiratory depression

4. Therapeutic effects of benzodiazepines usually occur in
    a. 24 hours
    b. 48 hours
    *c. 2 to 3 days
    d. 5 to 7 days

5. Buspirone (BuSpar) is unique from other antianxiety drugs in that it has
    a. muscle relaxant effects
    b. anticonvulsant effects
    *c. no propensity to cause physical dependence
    d. sedative effects

6. Used preoperatively, hydroxyzine (Vistaril) minimizes
    *a. anxiety, nausea, and vomiting
    b. oral secretions
    c. hypotension and bradycardia
    d. confusion

7. An antihistamine used as a hypnotic is
    a. zolpidem (Ambien)
    *b. diphenhydramine (Benadryl)
    c. flurazepam (Dalmane)
    d. chloral hydrate

8. Persons with the following disorder(s) should avoid sedative-hypnotics:
    a. neurological disease
    *b. end-stage renal disease
    c. endocrine disorders
    d. heart disease

9. Prior to the administration of hypnotics, the nurse should assess the client for
    a. agitation
    *b. drug dependence and abuse
    c. anorexia
    d. heart disease

10. Flumazenil (Romazicon), an antidote for benzodiazepine toxicity, can cause
    *a. agitation, confusion, and seizures
    b. cerebral hemorrhage and dystonia
    c. hypertension and renal insufficiency
    d. hypotension, dysrhythmias, and cardiac arrest

11. You know that your teaching has been effective if a client who is taking a benzodiazepine states,

    a. "I can only take the medication with meals."

    *b. "I know this drug needs to be gradually tapered before discontinuation."

    c. "I cannot take this medication if I am using aspirin."

    d. "I will take this medication for the rest of my life."

12. Clients taking benzodiazepines are at higher risk for toxicity if this level is low:

    a. calcium

    *b. albumin

    c. potassium

    d. bicarbonate

CHAPTER 9

1. Thorazine (chlorpromazine) and Compazine (prochlorperazine) can also be used for

    a. pain

    b. hypertension

    *c. intractable hiccups

    d. seizures

2. During the initial phase of therapy with psychotherapeutic drugs

    a. a loading dose is administered over a 72-hour period, then the drug dosage is slowly reduced

    *b. a low therapeutic dose is given initially, then increased gradually until symptoms are eliminated or reduced

    c. a small dose is administered, then the drug dose is titrated upward

    d. a large dose is administered for 2 weeks, then the drug dosage is titrated downward

3. Negative symptoms of schizophrenia treated with neuroleptic drugs include

    a. insomnia

    b. hallucinations

    *c. blunted affect

    d. paranoia

4. Persons with psychosis exhibit

    *a. disorganized and often bizarre thinking

    b. slowed reaction time and poor coordination

    c. short manic episodes, followed by long depressive episodes

    d. short- and long-term memory deficits

5. Administration of all of the following drugs can result in psychosis except

    a. antidepressants

    *b. beta blockers

    c. anticonvulsants

    d. steroids

6. Phenothiazines can cause

    a. bradycardia

    b. bradypnea

    *c. hypotension

    d. hypoglycemia

7. Phenothiazines treat nausea and vomiting by blocking the following receptors:

    a. acetylcholine

    b. epinephrine

    *c. dopamine

    d. aspartate

8. The usual loading dose of chlorpromazine (Thorazine) for a psychiatric client with acute agitation is

    a. 25–50 mg/day

    b. 50–100 mg/day

    c. 200–400 mg/day

    *d. 400–1500 mg/day

9. An antipsychotic drug used for the treatment of Tourette's syndrome is

    a. chlorprothixene (Taractan)

    b. thiothixene (Navane)

    c. clozapine (Clozaril)

    *d. haloperidol (Haldol)

10. The use of antipsychotic drugs is contraindicated in the following conditions:

    a. renal insufficiency

    b. emphysema

    *c. parkinsonism

    d. migraine headaches

11. The following medication has fewer extrapyramidal effects and greater effectiveness in relieving negative symptoms of schizophrenia:
    a. chlorprothixene (Taractan)
    b. thiothixene (Navane)
    *c. clozapine (Clozaril)
    d. haloperidol (Haldol)

CHAPTER 10

1. The following is an anticholinergic response associated with antipsychotic drugs:
    a. blood dyscrasias
    b. lowered seizure threshold
    c. weight gain
    *d. urinary retention

2. Anticholinergic blockade by antidepressant drugs can result in the following symptom:
    *a. tachycardia
    b. tremors
    c. constipation
    d. erectile dysfunction

3. Fluoxetine hydrochloride (Prozac)
    *a. inhibits reuptake of serotonin
    b. blocks histamine
    c. prevents the reuptake of norepinephrine
    d. acts as an alpha-adrenergic blocker

4. A client is admitted to your unit because of a tricyclic antidepressant overdose. The following nursing diagnosis would be a priority:
    a. risk for injury related to sedation
    b. knowledge deficit related to effects and usage of antidepressants
    *c. respiratory failure related to CNS depression
    d. decreased cardiac output related to hypotension

5. Persons taking tricyclic antidepressants should
    *a. sit on the side of the bed for several minutes before getting up
    b. increase foods high in calcium in their diet
    c. elevate their legs whenever they sit down
    d. weigh themselves daily

6. The following medication, if administered concurrently with lithium, can produce a toxic effect:
    a. prednisone
    b. digoxin (Lanoxin)
    c. insulin
    *d. bumetanide (Bumex)

7. Clients taking an MAO inhibitor should be monitored frequently for
    *a. hypertension
    b. respiratory congestion
    c. decreased urinary output
    d. anemia

8. Your client is started on a tricyclic for depression. He should avoid the following because it will decrease his serum drug levels:
    a. caffeine
    *b. nicotine
    c. vitamin C
    d. red wine

9. Clients who are receiving bupropion (Wellbutrin) may develop CNS stimulation. Therefore, for the first few days of drug administration they may require a/an
    a. hypnotic
    *b. sedative
    c. anticonvulsant
    d. muscle relaxant

10. A therapeutic response from fluoxetine (Prozac) should be seen in
    a. 24–48 hours
    b. 7–10 days
    *c. 2–3 weeks
    d. 2–3 months

CHAPTER 11

1. Absence seizures are characterized by
    *a. alterations in consciousness that last seconds
    b. automatic and repetitive movements
    c. abnormal movements and bizarre behavior
    d. sustained contraction of skeletal muscle

2. AEDs control seizure activity by blocking the movements of
   a. potassium ions
   b. calcium ions
   c. chloride ions
   *d. sodium ions

3. The drug commonly used to prevent seizures in a person with a head injury is
   a. carbamazepine (Tegretol)
   b. valproic acid (Depakene)
   *c. phenytoin (Dilantin)
   d. phenobarbital

4. Abrupt withdrawal of antiseizure agents may precipitate
   a. hypertensive crisis
   b. cardiac dysrhythmias
   c. respiratory arrest
   *d. status epilepticus

5. The antiseizure drug used IV to terminate acute convulsive seizures is
   *a. lorazepam (Ativan)
   b. phenytoin (Dilantin)
   c. ethosuximide (Zarontin)
   d. gabapentin (Neurontin)

6. Phenobarbital has a long half-life; therefore, to reach therapeutic serum levels, it takes
   a. 1 week
   *b. 2–3 weeks
   c. 1 month
   d. 2–3 months

7. Valproic acid, an antiseizure drug, is also used for
   *a. manic reactions of bipolar disorder
   b. ADHD (attention-deficit hyperactivity disorder)
   c. Crohn's disease
   d. schizophrenia

8. In a person with a seizure disorder, all of the following may precipitate a seizure except
   a. ingestion of alcoholic beverages
   b. fever
   c. physical or emotional stress
   *d. strenuous exercise

9. Larger doses of antiseizure medications may be needed
   a. if the client has renal disease
   *b. in cases involving trauma
   c. if the client has liver disease
   d. in cases in which seizures occur before age 6

10. You know that your teaching regarding antiseizure medications has been effective if the client states "I will take the medication
    a. with 8 ounces of water."
    b. with fluids high in vitamin C."
    *c. with meals."
    d. on an empty stomach."

11. Mr. J is admitted with acute alcohol intoxication. Which medication may be administered as he undergoes alcohol withdrawal?
    a. primidone (Mysoline)
    b. ethosuximide (Zarontin)
    *c. clonazepam (Klonopin)
    d. phenytoin (Dilantin)

12. Mr. J's Dilantin level is 12 ug/mL. Based on this level you would
    *a. continue the dose as ordered
    b. decrease the daily dose
    c. hold the drug until further orders
    d. increase the daily dose

13. R. F. is to be sent home on Dilantin 100 mg b.i.d. Which of the following statements by R. F. lead you to believe he has understood your teaching?
    a. "I will take the medication on an empty stomach."
    b. "I will discontinue the drug immediately if any side effects occur."
    *c. "I will make routine visits to the dentist."
    d. "I will weigh myself daily."

14. An adverse effect of the administration of antiseizure medication is:
    *a. folic acid deficiency
    b. bradycardia
    c. increased appetite
    d. double vision

15. You are writing a nursing outcome for T. J., who has partial seizures and is receiving primidone (Mysoline). Which of the following would be appropriate? T. J. will experience

    *a. control of partial seizures

    b. minimal drug side effects

    c. seizure control without medications

    d. no further seizure activity

16. A client taking phenytoin (Dilantin) should be advised to

    a. have renal function studies once a month

    b. ingest daily large amounts of fluids high in vitamin C

    *c. brush and floss teeth frequently

    d. elevate the feet because swelling of the feet and ankles is a normal side effect of the medication

CHAPTER 12

1. Parkinsonism, which may occur with long-term use of antipsychotics, can be treated with

    *a. anticholinergic agents

    b. MAO inhibitors

    c. synthetic antiviral agents

    d. dopaminergic drugs

2. When teaching clients about anticholinergic antiparkinson drugs, it is important to instruct the client to avoid the concurrent use of

    a. aspirin compounds

    *b. antihistamines

    c. alcohol

    d. antianginal agents

3. A medication frequently used with levodopa because it enables more levodopa to reach the brain is

    a. bromocriptine (Parlodel)

    *b. carbidopa (Lodosyn)

    c. amantadine (Symmetrel)

    d. trihexyphenidyl (Artane)

4. The following statement by your client, who is taking amantadine hydrochloride (Symmetrel), leads you to believe that she needs additional teaching:

    a. "This drug is also used to treat viral infections."

    b. "This drug can accumulate if one has decreased renal function."

    *c. "My tremor and rigidity will improve in about 3 weeks after I begin this medication."

    d. "This drug is not effective for long term use."

5. The following vitamin should be avoided when a client is receiving levodopa:

    a. B_1 (thiamine)

    *b. B_6 (pyridoxine)

    c. B_2 (riboflavin)

    d. C (ascorbic acid)

6. When selegiline (Eldepryl) is administered, the nurse should assess for

    a. irregular heart rate

    *b. elevated blood pressure

    c. decreased urinary output

    d. gingival hyperplasia

7. A common adverse effect of anticholinergic agents used for the treatment of Parkinson's disease includes

    a. blood dyscrasias

    b. hypotension

    *c. urinary retention

    d. diarrhea

8. For which of the following conditions would an anticholinergic agent be contraindicated?

    a. first-degree heart block

    b. diabetes mellitus

    *c. glaucoma

    d. hypertension

9. Elderly persons using anticholinergic medications should avoid

    *a. strenuous exercise in high environmental temperatures

    b. fluids high in potassium

    c. foods high in vitamin K

    d. anything containing red dye

10. Elderly clients can have hallucinations when the following antiparkinson medications are administered:
    a. anticholinergic drugs
    b. MAO inhibitors
    c. COMT inhibitors
    *d. dopamine agonist drugs

11. A physician should be notified if the client develops the following side effect while on levodopa (Dopar):
    a. nausea and vomiting
    b. blurred vision
    *c. tachycardia
    d. edema

CHAPTER 13

1. Adverse reactions seen in individuals taking large doses of centrally acting muscle relaxants include
    a. muscle spasms
    b. insomnia
    *c. hypotension
    d. depression

2. Administration of muscle relaxants may result in
    a. anorexia
    b. elevated creatinine levels
    c. difficulty swallowing
    *d. elevated pulse rate

3. The only muscle relaxant that acts peripherally on the muscle itself is
    a. methocarbamol (Robaxin)
    b. diazepam (Valium)
    c. baclofen (Lioresal)
    *d. dantrolene (Dantrium)

4. Muscle spasms can be decreased by muscle relaxants and the concurrent use of
    a. anti-inflammatory drugs
    *b. massage
    c. steroids
    d. passive range of motion

5. Administered intravenously, this drug may be used to treat muscle spasms:
    a. metaxalone (Skelaxin)
    b. carisoprodol (Soma)
    c. baclofen (Lioresal)
    *d. methocarbamol (Robaxin)

6. The following lab study should be assessed before dantrolene (Dantrium) is administered:
    a. serum glucose and creatinine
    b. serum potassium and sodium
    c. lipase and amylase
    *d. AST and ALT

7. Persons using skeletal muscle relaxants should avoid
    *a. alcohol
    b. high-protein foods
    c. caffeine
    d. nicotine

8. Before administering an IV muscle relaxant, you should inform the client that he or she may experience transient
    a. inability to swallow
    *b. blurred vision and flushing
    c. palpitations
    d. nausea and vomiting

CHAPTER 14

1. Adverse effects of propofol (Diprivan) include
    a. increased risk of laryngospasm
    b. severe nausea and vomiting
    c. increased tracheobronchial secretions
    *d. hypotension and apnea

2. Nitrous oxide is used alone for
    *a. dental procedures
    b. diagnostic procedures
    c. analgesia
    d. major surgical procedures

3. A local anesthetic used for epidural infusion is
    a. procaine (Novocaine)
    *b. lidocaine (Xylocaine)
    c. butamben (Batesin)
    d. mepivacaine(Carbocaine)

4. Anticholinergic drugs are used preoperatively to prevent
    a. postoperative hypotension
    b. urination during surgery
    c. bradycardia
    *d. excessive oral secretions

5. Injection of the anesthetic solution around the area to be anesthetized refers to
    a. peripheral nerve block
    *b. field block anesthesia
    c. infiltration
    d. surface anesthesia

6. Lidocaine is contraindicated for topical use in persons
    *a. with abraded skin or mucous membranes
    b. who are febrile
    c. with peripheral vascular disease
    d. who are using anticoagulants

CHAPTER 15

1. Persons routinely using opioids will experience the following adverse effect:
    a. anxiety
    b. bradycardia
    *c. constipation
    d. bradypnea

2. Alcohol withdrawal treatment is focused on preventing
    a. bradycardia
    b. hypotension
    *c. seizures
    d. gastrointestinal bleeding

3. When administering drugs to alcoholic patients, you should avoid
    *a. elixirs
    b. magmas
    c. syrups
    d. lozenges

4. Persons receiving flumazenil (Romazicon) for benzodiazepine overdose must be closely observed because the drug may
    a. cause sedation and respiratory depression
    b. induce acute tubular necrosis
    *c. precipitate acute withdrawal symptoms
    d. cause severe nausea and vomiting

5. An antihypertensive drug sometimes used to relieve withdrawal symptoms is
    a. atenolol (Tenormin)
    b. methyldopa (Aldomet)
    *c. clonidine (Catapres)
    d. guanethidine (Ismelin)

6. All of the following are drugs used in drug treatment to reduce preoccupation with drug use except
    a. methadone
    b. LAAM (Orlaam)
    c. naltrexone (ReVia)
    *d. chlordiazepoxide (Librium)

7. Persons receiving naltrexone (ReVia) should stop taking the drug at least _____ before a scheduled procedure:
    a. 24 hours
    b. 48 hours
    *c. 72 hours
    d. 2 weeks

8. The following group of chemicals is referred to as "uppers" and produces CNS stimulation:
    *a. amphetamines
    b. benzodiazepines
    c. heroin
    d. alcohol

9. Overdosage of cocaine can cause
   a. severe hemorrhaging of the nasal passages
   b. permanent lung damage
   *c. life-threatening cardiac arrhythmias
   d. anaphylactic reactions

10. The following disorder is associated with nicotine dependence:
   a. anorexia
   b. bradycardia
   c. constipation
   *d. depression

11. Before Mrs. J stops smoking, you should inform her about the signs and symptoms of withdrawal, which include
   *a. anxiety, irritability, and difficulty concentrating
   b. muscle cramping and palpitations
   c. chronic fatigue and food intolerance
   d. diarrhea, dehydration, and electrolyte imbalance

12. Transdermal patches that produce a steady blood level of nicotine are contraindicated in persons with
   *a. angina pectoris or dysrhythmias
   b. renal insufficiency or hepatitis
   c. chronic lung disease
   d. diabetes mellitus

13. Inhaled substances containing gasoline, benzene, or carbon tetrachloride can cause serious damage to the
   a. lungs, pancreas, and brain
   b. immune system and lymphatic system
   *c. liver, kidneys, and bone marrow
   d. mucous membranes, eyes, and thyroid gland

14. All of the following are appropriate for a client undergoing drug withdrawal; which one takes priority?
   a. ineffective individual coping related to reliance on alcohol or other drugs
   *b. risk for injury: adverse drug effects
   c. altered nutrition: less than body requirements related to drug effects and drug-seeking behavior
   d. altered thought processes related to the use of psychoactive drugs

CHAPTER 16

1. An expected outcome after the administration of methylphenidate (Ritalin) is
   a. elimination of behavioral problems
   *b. decreased hyperactivity
   c. increased intellectual capacity
   d. improvement of fine motor skills

2. The following statement by the parents of a child receiving methylphenidate indicates that they understand how the drug is to be used:
   a. "I know that my child can develop a tolerance to the medication, so we will monitor him."
   *b. "We will monitor his height and his weight."
   c. "Self-image and learning ability may diminish with the use of this drug."
   d. "Stimulants used for ADHD always produce a therapeutic effect."

3. Persons receiving methylphenidate for narcolepsy should be taught to avoid foods containing
   a. tyramine
   b. sodium
   *c. caffeine
   d. red dye

4. Your client, who is taking an amphetamine for narcolepsy, should be instructed to report the following adverse effect of the medication:
   a. increased motor activity
   b. decreased appetite
   *c. rapid heart rate
   d. constipation

5. Caffeine is added to ergot alkaloid to treat
   a. apnea
   b. insomnia
   *c. migraine headaches
   d. respiratory congestion

6. Doxapram (Dopram) increases
   *a. tidal volume and respiratory rate
   b. oxygen consumption
   c. oxygen production
   d. cardiac and urinary output

7. Caffeine is added to non-prescription analgesic preparations such as Excedrin to increase their
   *a. analgesic effect
   b. bronchodilator effect
   c. stimulant effect
   d. decongestant effect

CHAPTER 17

1. A side effect of nonselective beta-adrenergic blockers is
   a. increased heart rate
   *b. bronchoconstriction
   c. decreased gastric motility
   d. pupillary constriction

2. Cholinergic drugs can produce the following side effect:
   *a. bradycardia
   b. tachycardia
   c. constipation
   d. increased platelet aggregation

3. Adrenergic drugs may cause the following side effect:
   a. bronchoconstriction
   b. vasodilation
   *c. tachycardia
   d. diarrhea

4. One of the physiologic effects of the release of acetylcholine is
   *a. miosis
   b. mydriasis
   c. tachycardia
   d. constipation

5. Beta-adrenergic blockers are used for the treatment of
   a. asthma
   *b. angina
   c. anorexia
   d. alopecia

6. Anticholinergic drugs can produce the following side effect:
   a. bradycardia
   *b. tachycardia
   c. vasodilation
   d. diarrhea

7. When cholinergic drugs are administered, the nurse should observe the client for which one of the following adverse effects?
   a. vasoconstriction
   *b. bronchoconstriction
   c. fluid retention
   d. constipation

8. The following assessment is directly related to the stimulation of the parasympathetic nervous system:
   a. increased heart rate
   b. increased respiratory rate
   c. cold, clammy skin
   *d. constricted pupils

9. An expected outcome of the administration of adrenergic agents is
   a. urinary frequency
   b. vasodilation
   *c. bronchodilation
   d. bradycardia

CHAPTER 18

1. The use of isoproterenol (Isuprel) is contraindicated in persons with the following condition:
   a. diabetes mellitus
   *b. tachycardia
   c. hypotension
   d. bronchoconstriction

2. An expected outcome after the administration of a vasopressor, related to increased perfusion, is
   *a. increased urinary output
   b. headache
   c. flushing of the head and neck
   d. rapid respirations

3. The drug of choice for treating shock due to an anaphylactic reaction is
   a. isoproterenol (Isuprel)
   b. dopamine (Intropin)
   c. dobutamine (Dobutrex)
   *d. epinephrine (Adrenalin)

4. Adrenergic drugs are used for the treatment of
   a. heart failure
   *b. asthma
   c. tachycardia
   d. renal failure

5. Prolonged use of high doses of dopamine (Intropin), a vasopressor, may result in
   a. myocardial infarction secondary to arterial embolization
   b. angina secondary to vasospasm
   c. seizures secondary to diminished blood supply to the brain
   *d. gangrene secondary to peripheral vasoconstriction

6. The most common route for administering epinephrine (Adrenalin) is
   a. oral
   b. intramuscular
   *c. intravenous
   d. subcutaneous

7. Which of the following comments by Mr. J.'s wife leads you to believe that she has a good understanding of why her husband is receiving dobutamine (Dobutrex). The doctor ordered the medication to
   *a. "increase the force of the contraction of my husband's heart."
   b. "increase my husband's heart rate."
   c. "improve his peripheral circulation"
   d. "decrease his blood pressure."

8. Mr. J. was given epinephrine (Adrenalin) for hypotension and bradycardia. The physician now orders dopamine (Intropin). What will you do?
   a. refuse to give the medication
   *b. administer the medication as ordered
   c. schedule the medication for 4 hours after the administration of the adrenaline

d. give only a portion of the dose and observe for side effects; if no side effects occur, give the remainder of the dose

9. After a breathing treatment with isoproterenol (Isuprel), your client calls you into the room to show you her sputum and states, "I'm getting worse. Look, I have blood in my sputum." Your best response would be
   a. "The pink color is due to the irritation in your throat caused by coughing."
   b. "I will contact your physician and send a sputum specimen."
   *c. "It is common for the sputum to turn pink when isoproterenol (Isuprel) is given by inhalation. It is not blood."
   d. "You have no need to be alarmed. Increase your fluid intake and it will go away."

10. If the following drugs are administered concurrently with adrenergic drugs, they will increase adrenergic effects:
    a. beta-adrenergic blockers
    *b. xanthines
    c. anticholinergics
    d. antipsychotics

CHAPTER 19

1. The following medication would be beneficial for treating both angina and hypertension:
   a. metoprolol (Lopressor)
   b. pindolol (Visken)
   c. esmolol (Brevibloc)
   *d. atenolol (Tenormin)

2. The nurse should monitor clients receiving beta-adrenergic blocking agents for
   a. transient hypertension
   b. angina
   *c. heart failure
   d. urinary retention

3. Adverse reactions to beta-adrenergic blockers that the nurse should make the client aware of before discharge include
   a. headaches
   b. blurred vision
   c. confusion
   *d. hypotension

4. Nonselective beta-blockers used for the treatment of hypertension block
   a. beta$_1$-adrenergic receptors
   b. alpha-receptors
   *c. beta$_1$-adrenergic receptors and beta$_2$-adrenergic receptors
   d. beta$_1$-adrenergic receptors, beta$_2$-adrenergic receptors, and alpha receptors

5. Information the nurse should be aware of before administering a beta-adrenergic blocker includes the client's
   *a. pulse and blood pressure
   b. weight
   c. serum albumin level
   d. serum sodium and potassium levels

6. The following statement by a client receiving metoprolol (Lopressor) would lead you to believe that he needs additional instruction:
   a. "If I have side effects from the medication, I will contact my physician before I stop taking it."
   *b. "I will check my pulse daily and report it if it is under 50."
   c. "I will take the medication on an empty stomach."
   d. "I will report a weight gain of two pounds or more in 1 week."

7. Mr. J. was admitted to your unit with angina and was started on nadolol (Corgard). After 4 days, Mr. J. states he hasn't slept in days and has been having nightmares when he closes his eyes. Your best response to Mr J. would be
   *a. "I will contact the doctor and make him aware of your insomnia and nightmares."
   b. "These are common side-effects and they will get better the longer you are on the medication."
   c. "These symptoms are probably due to sleeping in a strange place. Once you get home, you will be able to sleep."
   d. "If your nightmares don't go away in 2 weeks, your doctor will stop the medication."

8. Mr. B. has all of the following diagnoses. Which one would you make the physician aware of before starting a beta-adrenergic blocker?
   a. hypertension
   b. angina

*c. asthma
   d. migraine headaches

9. The nurse will know that diltiazem (Cardizem) has been effective in treating a client with Raynaud's disease if the client experiences increased
   a. reflexes of the extremity
   b. movement
   *c. temperature of the extremity
   d. blood pressure in the extremity

10. The nurse will know that timolol (Timoptic) has been effective if the client's
    a. blood pressure is reduced
    *b. intraocular pressure is reduced
    c. pulse is reduced
    d. angina is reduced

11. The following behaviors by Mr. B., who is receiving atenolol (Tenormin) for hypertension, indicate successful teaching:
    a. using ibuprofen (Motrin) instead of aspirin
    b. drinking eight glasses of water daily
    c. eating foods high in roughage
    *d. taking pulse rate daily

12. The following beta-adrenergic blocking agent is effective in preventing migraine headaches:
    *a. propranolol (Inderal)
    b. nadolol (Corgard)
    c. timolol (Blocadren)
    d. acebutolol (Sectral)

13. An expected outcome of the administration of beta-adrenergic blocking agents is
    a. increased glucose production
    b. decreased cardiac perfusion
    *c. decreased cardiac output
    d. increased oxygen consumption

14. Mr. C. is receiving acebutolol (Sectral) for multifocal premature ventricular contractions. It is important to assess Mr. C's pulse rate as well as his
    a. breath sounds
    *b. blood pressure
    c. blood sugar
    d. orientation

15. The following statement by your client leads you to believe that she understands the teaching that you have done regarding nadolol (Corgard):

    *a. "If I experience side effects, I will not stop the medication."

    b. "I am not allowed to have any caffeine."

    c. "Smoking will not reduce the effectiveness of the medication."

    d. "I must have my blood pressure taken daily."

16. The following drug, when administered with propranolol (Inderal), will increase the effect of Inderal:

    a. atropine

    *b. digoxin (Lanoxin)

    c. isoproterenol (Isuprel)

    d. levarterenol (Levophed)

17. In reviewing Mr. J's history, you discover that he has a history of depression, myocardial infarction, peripheral vascular disease, and hypothyroidism. Which one of these diagnoses would you discuss with the physician before administering a beta-adrenergic blocker?

    a. myocardial infarction

    b. peripheral vascular disease

    *c. depression

    d. thyrotoxicosis

CHAPTER 20

1. Your client, who has been receiving bethanechol (Urecholine) for 1 week, develops sweating, flushing, abdominal cramps, and nausea. A possible explanation for the appearance of these symptoms is

    a. myasthenic crisis

    *b. cholinergic overdose

    c. anaphylactic reaction

    d. pulmonary edema

2. A cholinergic drug used for the treatment of Alzheimer's disease is

    a. bethanechol (Urecholine)

    b. neostigmine (Prostigmin)

    *c. tacrine (Cognex)

    d. physostigmine salicylate (Antilirium)

3. You will know that your client has myasthenia gravis if the client exhibits the following within 30 minutes after the administration of edrophonium (Tensilon):

    *a. increased muscle strength

    b. decreased adventitious breath sounds

    c. decreased muscle spasms

    d. increased urinary output

4. After receiving bethanechol (Urecholine), Mr. G's pulse drops from 80 to 70. You should

    a. contact the physician immediately

    *b. know that a drop in pulse rate is common with this drug

    c. check his pulse every hour for the next 24 hours

    d. have Mr. G. walk in the hall for 30 minutes, then recheck his pulse

5. Mr. J. is receiving a cholinergic agent and his pulse drops to 50. The treatment of choice for bradycardia is to administer a/an

    *a. anticholinergic drug

    b. antihistamine

    c. adrenergic blocking agent

    d. vasopressor

6. The nurse knows that the client has understood her teaching about bethanechol (Urecholine) if he states

    *a. "I will take the medicine before meals."

    b. "I must drink plenty of fluids to prevent constipation."

    c. "I must eat 6 small meals a day."

    d. "I will take a stool softener with the Urecholine."

7. You are admitting Mr. B. to the unit. The physician has ordered bethanechol (Urecholine) for urinary retention. Which of the following is a common adverse response to the medication?

    a. elevated serum calcium levels

    b. hypotension and bradycardia

    *c. nausea, vomiting, and diarrhea

    d. headaches

8. Mrs. P., with myasthenia gravis, is to receive pyridostigmine (Mestinon) at bedtime. Mrs. P. asks you why she must take the medication at bedtime. Your best reply is

    a. "You will have fewer side effects if you take the drug this way."

b. "By taking the medicine at night, it minimizes your secretions in the morning."

c. "By taking the drug, skin rashes are less likely to occur."

*d. "If you take the drug at bedtime, you will be better able to move about when you awaken."

9. Which of the following cholinergic drugs is the drug of choice for "atropine poisoning?"

a. bethanechol (Urecholine)

b. neostigmine (Prostigmin)

c. edrophonium (Tensilon)

*d. physostigmine salicylate (Antilirium)

CHAPTER 21

1. The physician has ordered a scopolamine patch for motion sickness for Mrs. Z. Which statement by Mrs. Z. leads you to believe she knows how to use the patch?

a. "I will place it on my chest each morning after I shower."

b. "I will use it only if I feel sick to my stomach."

c. "I will change the patch every 4 hours. I can use the patches for 1 week."

*d. "I will change the patch every 3 days."

2. Which of the following drugs may be used for initial treatment of parkinsonism?

a. flavoxate (Urispas)

b. benztropine (Cogentin)

*c. trihexyphenidyl (Artane)

d. oxybutynin (Ditropan)

3. The physician orders preoperative medications glycopyrrolate (Robinul) 1 mg and meperidine (Demerol) 50 mg IM. Before administering these medications, you should assess your client for the following disorder:

a. tachycardia

*b. glaucoma

c. hypertension

d. diabetes mellitus

4. After surgery, Mrs. A., who received glycopyrrolate (Robinul) and meperidine (Demerol) preoperatively, complains of mouth dryness. A teaching response to her would be :

a. "This is caused by your preoperative medication, which decreased your salivation. It is only temporary and will improve."

*b. "This is caused by loss of body fluid, which is induced by glycopyrrolate (Robinul)."

c. "You are probably dehydrated. The IV fluids you are receiving will correct the problem."

d. "Do not worry about it, the dryness will go away."

5. Atropine is prescribed to treat:

a. blurred vision

*b. bradycardia

c. paralytic ileus

d. urinary retention

6. Persons taking anticholinergic medications should be instructed to eat foods that are

a. high in protein

b. low in fat

*c. high in fiber

d. low in sodium

7. Anticholinergics

*a. inhibit gastric motility and secretions

b. stimulate the release of acetylcholine

c. increase respiratory tract secretions

d. increase secretion of sweat glands

8. Anticholinergic drugs are given to paraplegics to:

a. increase peristalsis

*b. increase bladder capacity

c. prevent vagal stimulation

d. reduce respiratory secretions

9. Mr. J., age 75, is started on flavoxate (Urispas) to relieve dysuria and urgency. One of the adverse effects of anticholinergics that he should be made aware of includes

a. skin rash

b. headache

c. weight gain

*d. blurred vision

10. Older adults using anticholinergic drugs are susceptible to:

  *a. heat stroke related to decreased perspiration

  b. diarrhea related to increased peristalsis

  c. frequency related to the diuretic effect of the medication

  d. hypotension related to increased sympathetic response

CHAPTER 22

1. The major organs of the endocrine system include all of the following except

  a. hypothalamus

  b. pituitary

  c. thyroid

  *d. gallbladder

2. The hormone produced by the kidneys that stimulates the bone marrow to produce red blood cells is

  a. prostaglandin

  b. leukotriene

  c. cytokine

  *d. erythropoietin

3. The connecting link between the nervous system and the endocrine system is the

  *a. hypothalamus

  b. thalamus

  c. medulla oblongata

  d. posterior pituitary

4. Hormones that are secreted in circadian cyclic patterns include

  a. estrogen and progestin

  *b. ACTH and cortisol

  c. gastrin and secretin

  d. insulin and erythropoietin

5. The lipid-soluble steroid and thyroid hormones have a longer duration of action because they are

  a. inactivated by enzymes

  b. excreted in bile or urine

  *c. bound to plasma proteins

  d. inactivated by enzymes at receptor sites

6. A strong vasoconstrictor that participates in control of arterial blood pressure is

  a. adenyl cyclase

  b. somatostatin

  c. calcitonin

  *d. angiotensin II

7. Hyperfunction of an endocrine gland can be caused by

  a. inadequate blood flow

  *b. hormone-producing tumor

  c. aging

  d. inadequate protein synthesis

8. Mineralocorticoids help regulate electrolyte balance by

  a. enhancing excretion of sodium and water

  *b. promoting sodium retention and potassium loss

  c. stimulating release of ADH

  d. provoking the release of other hormones

9. ADH secreted by the posterior pituitary

  a. exerts anti-inflammatory effects

  b. suppresses fluid balance

  *c. maintains fluid balance

  d. enhances urinary excretion

10. A hormone that regulates the metabolic rate and influences growth and development is

  a. PTH or parathormone

  *b. T4 or thyroxine

  c. cortisol

  d. insulin

11. Insulin

  a. raises blood glucose levels by promoting hepatic glycogenolysis

  *b. is necessary for growth and development in children

  c. regulates osmolality of extracellular fluid

  d. is necessary for protein metabolism

12. The thyroid hormone

  a. promotes potassium retention and sodium excretion

  *b. regulates metabolism of glucose, lipids, and proteins

  c. regulates calcium and phosphorus metabolism

  d. promotes carbohydrate storage and protein catabolism

13. Corticosteroids are administered for the treatment of
    a. adrenal hypersecretion
    b. extravasation of chemotherapy agents
    c. impaired development of secondary sex characteristics
    *d. inflammatory processes

14. The following disease is treated with adrenal corticosteroids:
    *a. Addison's disease
    b. anorexia
    c. Cushing's disease
    d. hyperthyroidism

15. Persons receiving corticosteroids need to be monitored for decreases in
    a. weight
    *b. potassium levels
    c. blood pressure
    d. red blood cell production

16. When an individual is placed in a stressful situation, increased amounts of the following hormone will be excreted:
    *a. epinephrine
    b. insulin
    c. estrogen
    d. thyroxine

17. Mrs. J. is admitted with elevated blood sugar, weakness, and irritability. Based on Mrs. J's symptoms, the nurse would suspect an abnormality in which of the following endocrine glands?
    a. adrenal
    b. thyroid
    *c. pancreas
    d. parathyroid

18. A 6-year-old is diagnosed with hypothyroidism. Her physician prescribes thyroid hormone replacement because an adequate thyroid level is necessary for
    *a. regulation of metabolism and growth and development
    b. regulation of calcium and phosphate metabolism
    c. development of most secondary sexual characteristics
    d. regulation of sodium and potassium balance

19. ADH is secreted by the body to control
    a. blood volume
    b. serum glucose levels
    *c. osmolarity of body fluids
    d. serum calcium levels

20. Glucocorticoids influence
    a. potassium retention and sodium loss
    b. metabolism of glucose, lipids, and proteins
    c. the development of feminine characteristics
    *d. carbohydrate storage and protein catabolism

21. The gastrointestinal mucosa secretes which of the following hormones that is important in the digestive process?
    a. liothyronine
    *b. cholecystokinin
    c. tetraiodothyronine
    d. prolactin

22. Mr. P. is an insulin-dependent diabetic who is started on Synthroid. The addition of Synthroid
    a. will have no effect on his insulin requirements
    *b. may increase his insulin requirements
    c. may decrease his insulin requirements
    d. is likely to cause a toxic effect that must be carefully assessed for

CHAPTER 23

1. The following hormone stimulates the adrenal cortex to produce adrenocorticosteroids:
   *a. corticotropin
   b. estrogen
   c. thyroxine
   d. oxytocin

2. FSH does all of the following except
   a. stimulate the production and growth of sperm
   *b. stimulate secretion of male sex hormones
   c. act on the ovaries in a cyclical fashion
   d. stimulate growth of ovarian follicles

3. The following plays a part in milk production:
   a. thyrotropin
   *b. prolactin
   c. oxytocin
   d. melanocyte

4. The antidiuretic hormone ADH causes
   *a. reabsorption of water
   b. concentration of extracellular fluids
   c. elevation of osmotic pressure
   d. decreased arterial blood pressure

5. Nafarelin (Synarel) is used
   a. for women with hypothalamic amenorrhea
   b. in diagnostic tests of gonadotropic functions
   *c. in the treatment of endometriosis
   d. to induce ovulation

6. A medication administered subcutaneously to inhibit diarrhea in persons with carcinoid tumors, vasoactive intestinal peptide tumors, and AIDS is
   a. gonadorelin hydrochloride (Factrel)
   *b. octreotide (Sandostatin)
   c. nafarelin (Synarel)
   d. gonadorelin acetate (Lutrepulse)

7. A medication administered to stimulate synthesis of hormones by the adrenal cortex is
   a. cosyntropin (Cortrosyn)
   b. protirelin (Thypinone)
   *c. corticotropin (Acthar)
   d. gonadorelin hydrochloride (Factrel)

8. Somatropin (Humatrope), a growth hormone, must be administered to children before
   a. they start school
   b. full growth is achieved
   c. age 8
   *d. puberty

9. A woman receiving HCG (Follutein) should be instructed that she could experience the following adverse effects with prolonged use of this medication:
   *a. edema
   b. acne and weight gain
   c. hirsutism
   d. diabetes mellitus

10. Diabetes insipidus, caused by hypofunction of the posterior pituitary gland, is treated with
    a. dexamethasone (Decadron)
    *b. vasopressin (Pitressin)
    c. methylprednisolone (Solu-Medrol)
    d. physostigmine (Antilirium)

11. The physician orders 10 units of oxytocin (Pitocin) in 1000 mL of D5W (10 milliunits/mL). Using microdrip tubing (1 mL = 60 drops), how fast will you run the IV to administer 3 milliunits/minute?
    a. 12 drops/minute
    b. 14 drops/minute
    c. 16 drops/minute
    *d. 18 drops/minute

12. Menotropins (Pergonal) is used to
    a. promote development of secondary sex characteristics
    *b. induce ovulation
    c. promote bone growth
    d. treat diabetes insipidus

CHAPTER 24

1. Mr. T is to receive methylprednisolone sodium succinate (Solu-Medrol) intravenously for acute respiratory distress. If he has the following condition, you will use caution when administering the medication:
   a. coronary artery disease
   b. chronic lung disease
   *c. peptic ulcer disease
   d. urinary retention

2. A client with adult-onset diabetes, controlled by oral medication, is receiving a glucocorticoid; you should assess him for
   a. decreased blood glucose levels
   b. increased effect of hypoglycemic agent
   c. decreased effectiveness of Solu-Medrol
   *d. elevated blood glucose levels

3. D. A. has been on long-term steroid therapy and is admitted with exacerbation of nephrosis. The following objective sign is related to chronic steroid use:
   a. dry, flaky skin
   *b. weight gain
   c. tachycardia
   d. decreased night vision

4. Mrs. B, who has had steroid therapy twice a day for 1 year, is scheduled for surgery tomorrow and is to be NPO after midnight. You should anticipate the following:

a. reduction in steroid dosage before surgery

b. discontinuation of steroids until after surgery

*c. continuation of steroids despite surgery

d. elevation of dosages needed for pain relief

5. The following nursing diagnosis is most applicable for a client on long-term steroids:

*a. potential for infection

b. decreased cardiac output

c. ineffective airway clearance

d. alteration in temperature regulation

6. The following nursing measure is appropriate for a neurosurgical client receiving dexamethasone (Decadron):

a. withhold steroid if nauseated

b. force oral fluids

c. reduce protein intake

*d. check stools for occult blood

7. Your client is to be discharged. You instruct her that the reason prednisone is ordered every other day is to

a. eliminate side effects

b. prolong therapeutic effects

c. prevent steroid tolerance

*d. minimize adverse effects

8. Long-term ingestion of prednisone can result in

a. hyponatremia

b. hyperkalemia

*c. hypocalcemia

d. hyperchloremia

9. Insulin-dependent diabetic clients started on prednisone (Deltasone) may need to

a. decrease the amount of insulin they are taking

*b. increase the amount of insulin they are taking

c. keep the dosage of insulin the same

d. stop taking insulin while they are receiving the medication

10. To prevent osteoporosis, postmenopausal women receiving estrogen should

*a. exercise daily

b. take supplemental calcium concurrently

c. eat foods high in vitamin K

d. take the medication with antacids

11. Prednisone is administered to persons with nephrosis to

a. promote diuresis

b. prevent sodium retention

*c. reduce urinary protein loss

d. prevent urinary tract infection

12. When administering corticosteroid inhalers, you should instruct clients to

a. use the inhaler no more than once a day

b. decrease their sodium intake

*c. rinse their mouth after administration

d. increase their fluid intake

13. A client is started on 2 inhalers: beclomethasone (Vanceril) 2 puffs and albuterol (Proventil) 3 puffs t.i.d. You know that your teaching has been effective if he states, "I will

a. wait 5 minutes between each puff."

b. take these medications one hour before meals, for best effectiveness."

c. rinse my mouth before administering them."

*d. use the Proventil first, followed by the Vanceril."

CHAPTER 25

1. When assessing a client who is taking levothyroxine (Synthroid) for hyperthyroidism, the nurse would expect the following side effects:

*a. nervousness, tachycardia, tremors

b. somnolence, bradycardia, paresthesia

c. hyperglycemia, hypertension, edema

d. buffalo hump, constipation, sodium loss

2. The primary mode of action for propylthiouracil is to

a. destroy part of the thyroid gland

*b. inhibit production of thyroid hormone

c. suppress the anterior pituitary gland's hormonal secretions

d. sedate the CNS and suppress the cardiac function

3. A sign of hyperglycemia is

*a. tetany

b. lethargy

c. polyuria

d. flank pain

4. Weight loss, insomnia, and tachycardia are symptoms associated with
   a. chronic thyroiditis
   b. hyperglycemia
   c. hypothyroidism
   *d. hyperthyroidism

5. A person experiencing hypothyroidism may exhibit
   a. anemia
   b. hypotension
   c. elevated glucose levels
   *d. decreased cardiac output

6. A simple goiter results from the following deficiency:
   a. magnesium
   b. chloride
   *c. iodine
   d. copper

7. Antithyroid drugs are commonly administered for
   a. 1–2 months
   *b. 6 months to 2 years
   c. 2–5 years
   d. a lifetime

8. A client receiving propylthiouracil needs to be assessed for hypothyroidism, symptoms of which include
   *a. lethargy
   b. tachycardia
   c. fever
   d. weight loss

9. A 5 year old is diagnosed with hypothyroidism. If left untreated, the following may develop:
   *a. mental retardation
   b. renal dysfunction
   c. an immune deficiency
   d. paralytic ileus

10. Potassium iodide, used for the treatment of hyperthyroidism, is also used as
    a. a topical preparation for acne
    b. an antidysrhythmic
    *c. an expectorant
    d. a potassium supplement

CHAPTER 26

1. Calcium helps to regulate
   a. action potential of the heart
   b. blood coagulation and platelet adhesion
   c. the influx of sodium in excitable tissues
   *d. all of the above

2. A function of extracellular phosphorus is
   a. activation of B-complex vitamins
   *b. maintenance of acid–base balance
   c. carbohydrate metabolism
   d. regulation of cell membrane permeability

3. A complication of hypercalcemia is
   *a. decreased level of consciousness progressing to unresponsiveness
   b. muscle tetany progressing to seizures
   c. bradycardia progressing to cardiac failure
   d. numbness and tingling of the extremities

4. A biologic response to hypocalcemia is
   a. decreased nerve and muscle function
   *b. decreased clotting times
   c. increased bone density
   d. increased pulse rate

5. Long-term use of which of the following medications can lead to osteoporosis:
   a. beta-adrenergic blockers
   b. calcium channel blockers
   c. ACE inhibitors
   *d. corticosteroids

6. Your client is admitted for diabetic ketoacidosis. You should observe her for symptoms of
   a. hypokalemia
   b. hypocalcemia
   *c. hypercalcemia
   d. hyperphosphatemia

7. Calcitonin is used for clients with renal disease to
   a. prevent formation of renal calculi
   b. interfere with calcium metabolism
   *c. enhance renal excretion of calcium
   d. supplement existing supplies of calcium

8. Hypocalcemia must be assessed for after
   a. bowel resection
   b. neurosurgery
   c. open heart surgery
   *d. thyroidectomy

CHAPTER 27

1. A distinguishing characteristic of type 1 diabetes is that
   a. blood sugar can be controlled with diet
   *b. exogenous insulin is required for life
   c. oral agents can control the disease process
   d. it always starts in childhood

2. A client in diabetic ketoacidosis (DKA) with a blood sugar of 600 is to receive an initial dose of 25 U insulin IV. The type of insulin that will be administered is
   a. NPH insulin
   b. lente insulin
   c. ultralente insulin
   *d. regular insulin

3. A type 2 diabetic is switched from chlorpropamide (Diabinese) to glyburide (DiaBeta). The nurse should instruct the client that
   a. "It is less potent, so you will need to take a larger dose."
   *b. "It stimulates insulin production, so you need to eat soon after taking the medication."
   c. "It is more potent and longer lasting, so you should take it every other day."
   d. "The two medications are virtually the same."

4. When type 1 diabetics ingest alcohol in moderate amounts it will
   a. increase the blood sugar
   b. be absorbed more rapidly because of the diabetes
   c. increase the risk of vascular complications
   *d. decrease the blood sugar

5. The following information should be included when teaching a client about insulin administration:
   a. intermediate-acting insulin is clear in color
   b. insulin should be shaken well before drawing up the dose
   c. an air bubble should be placed in the syringe for proper dispersion of the insulin
   *d. when mixing regular and NPH insulin in the same syringe, draw up regular insulin first

6. A 6 year old, newly diagnosed with type 1 diabetes (IDDM), may be at high risk for
   a. sleep pattern disturbance
   b. anxiety
   c. self-care deficit
   *d. alteration in growth and development

7. The following can precipitate a hypoglycemic reaction in an insulin-dependent diabetic:
   a. drinking alcohol with a meal
   b. increasing the caloric intake
   c. decreasing the amount of daily exercise
   *d. eating meals at sporadic times

8. You should be aware that the following is a contraindication to metformin (Glucophage):
   a. reduced hemoglobin level
   b. elevated prothrombin time
   c. reduced calcium level
   *d. elevated creatinine level

9. You know that your teaching has been effective if your client, taking chlorpropamide (Diabinese), states
   *a. "I will report headache and feelings of lethargy promptly."
   b. "I will take the medication with an antacid."
   c. "Sporadic mealtimes are allowed with this agent."
   d. "Hypoglycemic reactions do not require treatment when using this drug."

10. Human insulin is recommended for the following clients except those with
    a. gestational diabetes
    b. type 2 diabetes controlled on oral antidiabetic agents with systemic infections
    c. type 1 diabetics who have had diabetes for numerous years
    *d. type 2 diabetes controlled by diet

11. The type of insulin that should be used in an insulin pump is
    a. NPH
    *b. regular
    c. semilente
    d. Lente

12. A client using an insulin pump should be instructed to monitor his blood glucose level a minimum of
    a. daily
    b. weekly
    c. twice a day
    *d. four time a day

13. The best indicator of overall diabetic control is
    a. fasting blood glucose levels
    b. 2-hour postprandial blood glucose levels
    c. absence of acetone in the urine
    *d. glycosylated hemoglobin levels

14. The following is a symptom of hyperglycemia when it occurs at night:
    a. nightmares
    b. cold, clammy sweat
    *c. nocturia
    d. a headache on awakening

CHAPTER 28

1. Persons using birth control pills are at risk for developing blood clots because estrogen
    a. increases serum triglycerides, cholesterol, and glucose
    b. stimulates skeletal growth causing increased production of RBCs
    *c. increases blood levels of several clotting factors
    d. causes peripheral vasoconstriction

2. Mr. B., a 76-year-old man, is started on estrogen for metastatic prostate cancer. Which of the following statements by Mr. B. leads you to believe that he needs further teaching?
    a. "The doctor will check my blood sugars on a routine basis."
    *b. "I may experience impotence, which will sub-side when the drug is stopped."

    c. "I will not become alarmed if my breasts enlarge."
    d. "I will take this medication for the rest of my life."

3. Mrs. K. is a 33-year-old mother of two with a history of asthma and migraine headaches. She is on a low-residue diet for colitis. Which of the factors in Mrs. K.'s history may contraindicate the use of birth control pills?
    *a. migraine headaches
    b. age
    c. asthma
    d. colitis

4. Estradiol (Estraderm) is administered to post-menopausal women to prevent
    a. endometriosis
    b. dysfunctional uterine bleeding
    *c. osteoporosis
    d. uterine cancer

5. Ms. H. is to be started on birth control pills. Which of the following statements indicates that she needs additional teaching?
    a. "I will monitor my weight and have my blood pressure checked monthly."
    b. "I will have a Pap smear done on a yearly basis."
    *c. "I will continue to do monthly self-breast examination even though these pills should decrease my risk for developing breast cancer."
    d. "I know nausea is common so I will make sure that I take the medication at the same time each day with food."

6. The following statements by your client leads you to believe that she has a good understanding of how to take Nelova 10/11:
    *a. "I will take the medication for 3 weeks and a placebo for a week."
    b. "I will take a pill every morning and evening."
    c. "If I miss a pill, I will not take two the next day."
    d. "If I experience break-through bleeding, I should immediately stop the medication."

7. The following medications, when administered concurrently with oral contraceptives, will decrease their effect:
    *a. anticonvulsants

b. antihypertensives

c. anticoagulants

d. anticholinergics

8. The following instructions should be included when you are teaching someone about transdermal estrogen:

    a. apply the patches to the chest and upper back only

    b. the patches are irritating, so apply a thin layer of medicated cream before application of the patch

    c. the patch should be applied in the morning and taken off at bedtime

    *d. change the patches every 7 days

9. Persons taking estrogen need to be assessed regularly for the following adverse effect:

    a. hypoglycemia

    b. weight loss

    *c. depression

    d. arrhythmias

CHAPTER 29

1. The following medications, if administered concurrently with anabolic steroids, will decrease their effect:

    a. beta-adrenergic blockers

    *b. antihistamines

    c. thiazide diuretics

    d. cholinergic drugs

2. Persons taking anabolic steroids may experience which of the following adverse effects?

    a. elevated BUN

    b. elevated blood sugar

    c. bradycardia

    *d. jaundice

3. Physical changes that occur with the use of anabolic steroids in males include

    a. thinning of skin

    b. hair loss

    *c. reduced sperm count

    d. increased endurance

4. When androgens are administered to adult females, the following can result

    a. atrophy of breasts

    b. rapid bone growth

    c. loss of pubic hair

    *d. suppression of menstruation

5. Nandrolone decanoate (Deca-Durabolin) may be administered to adult women to treat

    a. endometriosis

    b. fibrocystic breast disease

    c. postpartum breast engorgement

    *d. anemia associated with renal disease

6. Mr. J's physician starts him on androgens for treatment of impotence. Which of the following statements by Mr.J. leads you to believe that he has understood the teaching that you have done?

    a. "If I experience increasing baldness, I will contact my physician immediately."

    *b. "If my skin appears yellow or my urine turns dark, I will contact my physician."

    c. "I know that my red blood count may drop so I will look for bruising and contact my physician if I see any."

    d. "I know that headaches are common with this drug, so I will not become alarmed if I have a severe headache."

7. A client receiving methyltestosterone (Metandren) for advanced breast cancer should be assessed for the following electrolyte disturbances:

    a. hyponatremia

    b. hypokalemia

    *c. hypercalcemia

    d. hyperchloremia

8. When nandrolone phenpropionate (Durabolin) is ordered for the treatment of anemia, it should be given with

    *a. folic acid

    b. iron

    c. thiamine

    d. vitamin B_{12}

9. Use of high doses of anabolic steroids by a female can result in the following:

    *a. masculinization

    b. immobility of joints

    c. obesity

    d. hypertension

10. Changes that can occur in adult males with the use of androgens are
    a. enlargement of prostate
    b. hair loss
    *c. suppression of sex drive
    d. increase in height

11. Danazol (Danocrine) is administered to prevent
    a. folic acid deficiencies
    b. excessive blood loss during menstruation
    *c. fibrocystic breast disease
    d. toxic shock syndrome

12. An expected outcome when oxandrolone (Oxandrin) is administered for osteoporosis is an increase in
    a. sexual desire
    *b. tissue mass
    c. muscle strength
    d. exercise tolerance

13. Women receiving androgen treatment for breast cancer may have an increase in the following:
    a. sodium
    b. potassium
    c. chloride
    *d. calcium

14. Which of the following statements by J., who is on testosterone for cryptorchidism, leads you to believe that he has understood the teaching that you have done: "I may . . .
    *a. have increased body hair."
    b. have decreased sexual desire."
    c. have a higher voice."
    d. have clear and soft skin."

15. When fluoxymesterone (Halotestin) is administered to a young male for hypogonadism the expected result is
    *a. growth of sexual organs
    b. decreased skin thickness
    c. increased protein metabolism
    d. retention of potassium

CHAPTER 30

1. A 1000 mL of D5W provides approximately
    a. 100 calories
    *b. 170 calories
    c. 300 calories
    d. 500 calories

2. An electrolyte imbalance that can result from administering hypertonic sodium chloride solutions is
    a. hypokalemia
    b. hyperkalemia
    c. hyponatremia
    *d. hypernatremia

3. An expected outcome for Mr. C., who is being treated with IV fluids for severe dehydration, would be
    a. a drop in blood pressure
    *b. a drop in hematocrit
    c. an increase in serum sodium
    d. an increased serum potassium level

4. The following statement by your client would lead you to believe that she has understood the teaching that you have done about pancreatin, a pancreatic enzyme:
    a. "I will take the pancreatin on an empty stomach."
    b. "I will increase the fat in my diet."
    *c. "I will take the pancreatin with meals."
    d. "I will increase foods high in vitamin C in my diet."

5. Persons receiving anorexiant drugs to decrease appetite should be instructed that they are only effective for
    a. 1–2 weeks
    *b. 4–6 weeks
    c. 2–3 months
    d. 4–6 months

6. Phenylpropanolamine, an ingredient in Dexatrim, may produce the following:
    a. edema
    b. migraine headaches
    *c. hypertension
    d. diabetes mellitus

7. TPN (total parenteral nutrition)
   a. may cause a fluid deficit and metabolic acidosis
   b. provides essential fatty acids
   *c. provides carbohydrates and amino acids
   d. may lower serum sodium levels

8. Mr. J. is admitted from home with confusion. The following are the results of his blood studies: Na+ 118, K+ 3.5, glucose 80. After analyzing his blood study results, which electrolyte imbalance would you suspect is contributing to his confusion?
   *a. hyponatremia
   b. hypernatremia
   c. hypokalemia
   d. hypoglycemia

9. Mr. J., who has a 15-year history of COPD, is to receive Pulmocare for his supplemental feedings because
   a. it promotes healing
   *b. its metabolism produces less carbon dioxide
   c. it is high in nitrogen and high in carbohydrates
   d. it requires no digestion and leaves no fecal residue

CHAPTER 31

1. An example of a fat-soluble vitamin is
   a. pyridoxine (vitamin B_6)
   b. ascorbic acid (vitamin C)
   *c. vitamin E
   d. vitamin B_{12}

2. Vitamin D is used to treat
   a. hypercalcemia
   *b. hypocalcemia
   c. hyperparathyroidism
   d. hypomagnesemia

3. Vitamin E is necessary for
   *a. inhibition of hemolysis of red blood cells
   b. utilization of vitamin K
   c. production of prostaglandin
   d. metabolism of steroids

4. You need to inform a client about the following major side effect associated with the use of niacin:
   a. confusion
   b. fine motor tremor
   c. hypotension
   *d. intense flushing

5. To minimize unwanted side effects associated with niacin therapy, the client should be advised to take the following 30 minutes before each dose:
   a. Compazine
   b. acetaminophen
   *c. aspirin
   d. Senokot

6. The following statement by your client indicates an understanding about why the antilipemic therapy was ordered:
   a. "If I take this drug, I can eat whatever I want."
   *b. "I may need this medication for the rest of my life."
   c. "My urine will be clay-colored and have a pungent odor."
   d. "This drug will prevent me from having a stroke."

7. Persons who smoke cigarettes are at risk for developing a deficiency of which of the following vitamins?
   a. vitamin A
   b. vitamin B_6
   *c. vitamin C
   d. vitamin D

8. Mrs. J. has multiple sclerosis and has an indwelling catheter. Which of the following vitamins should you recommend that she take to acidify her urine and thereby help decrease her likelihood of developing a urinary tract infection?
   a. folic acid (folate)
   b. pantothenic acid (vitamin B_5)
   c. niacin (nicotinic acid)
   *d. vitamin C (ascorbic acid)

9. Persons taking oral contraceptives need to be instructed to increase the following vitamin in their diets:
   a. vitamin K
   *b. folic acid (Folate)
   c. vitamin D
   d. riboflavin (vitamin B_2)

10. Mrs. B. is started on vitamin B_{12} for pernicious anemia. An expected outcome of the administration of this medication is
    a. decreased bleeding
    *b. increased hematocrit
    c. decreased joint pain
    d. improved vision

11. Mr. H., a 59-year-old truck driver, is experiencing night blindness. An increase in which one of the following vitamins may help improve his vision?
    *a. vitamin A
    b. vitamin B_2
    c. vitamin C
    d. vitamin D

12. Mrs. J. is started on Coumadin and instructed to avoid foods high in vitamin K. These include
    a. carrots, potatoes, squash
    b. apricots, peaches, cantaloupe
    c. meat, whole milk, margarine
    *d. green leafy vegetables, wheat bran

13. Mrs. H. is experiencing lethargy, pallor, and dizziness. A deficit of which of the following vitamins can cause these symptoms?
    a. vitamin A
    *b. vitamin B_{12}
    c. vitamin C
    d. vitamin D

14. Mrs. C., who has pernicious anemia, asks you why vitamin B_{12} must be administered parenterally. The best response to her question is
    *a. the intrinsic factor in your stomach that is required for absorption of vitamin B_{12} is absent
    b. oral ingestion of vitamin B_{12} causes irritation and bleeding
    c. pernicious anemia causes changes in the mucous membrane lining and impairs absorption

d. with severe deficiencies like yours, oral vitamin B_{12} is not effective

15. Mr. C. complains of headaches, dizziness, insomnia, and depression. He may require supplementation of which of the following vitamins to correct these symptoms?
    a. pyridoxine (vitamin B_6)
    b. pantothenic acid (vitamin B_5)
    *c. niacin (vitamin B_3)
    d. riboflavin (vitamin B_2)

CHAPTER 32

1. The following statement by a client receiving potassium chloride (KCl) indicates that your teaching was effective:
   a. "If I get dizzy, I will stop taking the medication."
   *b. "I will take the medication with meals."
   c. "I must avoid citrus fruits."
   d. "I must decrease my fluid intake while taking this medication."

2. You should instruct a client receiving oral iron preparations about this potential side effect:
   a. clay-colored stools
   b. hypotension
   *c. constipation
   d. frequent flatus

3. You should teach clients to utilize the following food with iron, to enhance its absorption:
   *a. orange juice
   b. eggs
   c. bran
   d. mustard

4. The following outcome is indicative of successful treatment of anemia:
   a. elevated APTT
   *b. increased energy level
   c. decreased anxiety level
   d. decreased bilirubin levels

CHAPTER 33

1. All of the following factors predispose a person to infection except
   a. impaired blood supply
   *b. hypertension
   c. suppression of immune system
   d. advanced age

2. Some antimicrobial drugs work by
   a. enhancing cell metabolism and growth
   b. promoting protein synthesis
   *c. inhibiting cell wall synthesis
   d. stimulating bacterial reproduction

3. If your client has renal insufficiency, the dose of many antibiotics should be
   a. increased
   *b. decreased
   c. unchanged

4. An infection acquired in the hospital is referred to as a
   *a. nosocomial infection
   b. communal infection
   c. sustained infection
   d. antimicrobial infection

5. Most oral antimicrobials should be administered
   *a. 1 hour before meals
   b. with meals
   c. 1 hour after meals
   d. with a full glass of milk

6. A condition which can occur when the normal flora is disturbed during antibiotic therapy is known as
   a. organ toxicity
   *b. superinfection
   c. hypersensitivity
   d. allergic reaction

7. Antimicrobial medication is usually administered in the following way to treat a bacterial infection:
   *a. one drug is administered for a period of 7 to 10 days
   b. oral medications are administered for 3–4 weeks

c. two or more antibiotics are used at a time to prevent the development of resistance
   d. medications are not administered until the client experiences a temperature above 101 degrees F

8. When an antibiotic is chosen, the following must be taken into consideration:
   a. length of time the client has experienced symptoms
   *b. cultures and sensitivities which have been drawn
   c. the client's hydration status
   d. the client's age

9. Objective symptoms of infection include which of the following?
   a. lethargy
   b. anorexia
   *c. fever
   d. headache

10. You have just finished instructing your client on measures to help the body fight infections. Which of the following statements by your client would lead you to believe he needs additional instruction?
    a. "I will make sure I get adequate rest."
    b. "I know I must continue to eat and drink lots of fluids."
    c. "I will wash my hands."
    *d. "I will take my medicine until I no longer have a fever."

CHAPTER 34

1. Your client has had subacute bacterial endocarditis. His physician is likely to recommend
   *a. prophylactic use of penicillin prior to visiting the dentist
   b. low-dose penicillin therapy for the rest of his life
   c. doubling the recommended dose of penicillin if he undergoes a surgical procedure
   d. using only *Pseudomonas*-resistant antibodies

2. Penicillin may be the drug of choice for treating which of the following infections?

   *a. syphilis and gonorrhea

   b. vaginitis

   c. acne

   d. gastritis and pancreatitis

3. A broad-spectrum semisynthetic penicillin used to treat several gram-positive and gram-negative infections is

   a. dicloxacillin (Dynapen)

   b. nafcillin (Unipen)

   *c. ampicillin (Omnipen)

   d. methicillin (Staphcillin)

4. A penicillin used to treat *Pseudomonas* infections is

   a. cyclacillin (Cyclapen)

   b. amoxicillin (Augmentin)

   c. amoxicillin (Amoxil)

   *d. piperacillin (Pipracil)

5. Your client weighs 88 pounds and is to receive Unipen 50 mg/kg/day in 4 doses. How many milligrams should be given per dose?

   a. 250

   *b. 500

   c. 1000

   d. 2000

6. Probenecid (Benemid) is used with penicillin to

   *a. increase serum drug levels

   b. prevent an anaphylactic reaction

   c. break down the bacterial cell wall

   d. decrease the amount of penicillin needed for a therapeutic affect

7. Adverse effects of high-dose antibiotic therapy are

   *a. nausea, vomiting, diarrhea

   b. anorexia and weight loss

   c. constipation and fluid retention

   d. syncope, tachycardia, hypotension

NOTE: There are no questions for Chapter 35.

CHAPTER 36

1. Your health teaching for methenamine mandelate (Mandelamine) should include the following:

   *a. "Drink citrus juice with the medication to acidify the urine."

   b. "Take sodium bicarbonate with the medication to make the urine alkaline."

   c. "Limit your fluid intake to 3000 cc per day."

   d. "While you are taking this drug, limit your intake of foods high in sodium."

2. Phenazopyridine (Pyridium) is a urinary tract analgesic used to relieve which of the following symptoms?

   a. urinary retention

   b. hematuria

   *c. pain and urgency

   d. hesitancy

3. A client who has been started on sulfisoxazole (Gantrisin) should contact her physician if she experiences the following adverse effects:

   a. polydipsia

   b. tachycardia

   *c. hematuria

   d. dizziness

4. The following statement by Mr. P. leads you to believe that he understands the health teaching you have done about nitrofurantoin (Macrodantin):

   a. "I know that it will turn my urine blue-green."

   b. "I will take vitamin C along with the medication."

   *c. "I will take the medicine with food or milk."

   d. "I will take the medicine at bedtime so that it can dwell in my bladder."

5. Mrs. C. is started on trimethoprim (Proloprim) for a urinary tract infection. Prior to administering this drug, the nurse should assess the client for

   a. asthma

   b. hypertension

   c. diabetes mellitus

   *d. renal insufficiency

6. Mr. C. has just been started on sulfasalazine (Azulfidine) for ulcerative colitis. Mr. C. is also taking phenytoin (Dilantin) for control of epilepsy.

The nurse will monitor Mr. C. for potential drug interactions which could result in tolerance to

  a. increased toxicity of sulfonamides

  b. decreased therapeutic effectiveness of sulfon-amides

  *c. decreased renal clearance, therefore increased potential for renal toxicity

  d. increased risk of hepatotoxicity

7. Mr. J., a 79-year-old male, is started on sulfamethoxazole-trimethoprim (Bactrim) for a urinary tract infection; he should be observed for adverse effects which include

  a. liver toxicity

  *b. renal damage

  c. bone marrow depression

  d. congestive heart failure

8. A person receiving phenazopyridine (Pyridium) should be informed that it will change the color of urine to

  a. bluish-green

  *b. reddish-orange

  c. brown

  d. black

9. A measure that the nurse can encourage clients to use to reduce the risk of recurrent urinary tract infections is

  a. increase alkaline foods in your diet

  b. take tub baths, soaking 15 minutes daily

  c. use sterile gauze pads to cleanse after urinating

  *d. force fluids to 3000 cc daily

CHAPTER 37

1. Erythromycin is the drug of choice for treating

  *a. Legionnaire's disease

  b. bacterial endocarditis

  c. urinary tract infections

  d. acne

2. Erythromycin may be used with neomycin preoperatively to

  a. prevent pneumonia

  *b. suppress intestinal bacteria

  c. eliminate diphtheria

  d. treat diarrhea

3. It is recommended that erythromycin be administered

  a. with meals

  *b. on an empty stomach

  c. with milk an hour before meals or 2 hours after

  d. with crackers and no fluids to prevent nausea

4. Macrolides must be used with caution in clients who have

  a. renal disease

  *b. liver disease

  c. diabetes mellitus

  d. hypertension

5. The following medication, if administered with erythromycin, will increase the effect of the erythromycin

  a. penicillin

  b. tetracycline

  c. ampicillin

  *d. chloramphenicol (Chloromycetin)

6. Common side effects that occur after the administration of erythromycin include

  a. rash, fever, and itching

  b. urticaria and colitis

  *c. nausea, vomiting, and diarrhea

  d. shortness of breath

7. The following medications, if administered concurrently with erythromycin, will decrease its effects:

  *a. antacids

  b. beta-adrenergic blockers

  c. calcium channel blockers

  d. antidepressants

8. Erythromycin can be used as a substitute for penicillin to treat

  a. meningitis

  b. botulism

  c. chlamydial infections

  *d. syphilis

9. M. J., who weighs 44 pounds, is being treated with erythromycin ethylsuccinate (EES) for pneumonia. The recommended dose is 30/mg/kg/day. The medication is to be a administered q6h. How much medication should M. J. receive per dose?

    a. 100 mg

    b. 125 mg

    *c. 150 mg

    d. 175 mg

10. The dose of clarithromycin must be reduced if the client has preexisting

    a. heart failure

    b. respiratory disease

    *c. renal disease

    d. diabetes mellitus

CHAPTER 38

1. Your client, who is taking INH (Laniazid), rifampin (Rifadin), and pyrazinamide, calls you because her urine is orange-red. You tell her

    a. "You may be bleeding so you should see your doctor immediately."

    b. "This may be due to hepatic toxicity. You should discontinue the drugs."

    c. "You have a urinary tract infection; drink plenty of fluids."

    *d. "This is a normal response to rifampin."

2. Prior to initiating INH therapy, you should ask your client the following question:

    *a. "Are you pregnant?"

    b. "Are you allergic to aspirin?"

    c. "Do you have a family history of diabetes?"

    d. "Have you ever been hypertensive?"

3. Your client appears to have yellow sclerae. What other findings would lead you to believe that she may be experiencing hepatic toxicity from the antitubercular drugs?

    a. diarrhea

    b. numbness and tingling

    c. visual changes

    *d. clay-colored stools

4. The following drug should be taken with food to prevent nausea, vomiting, and diarrhea:

    a. rifampin (Rifadin)

    *b. para-amino salicylic acid (PAS)

    c. INH (Laniazid)

    d. streptomycin

5. Your client is receiving antitubercular drug therapy. You notice that her urinary output has dropped in the past week. Which lab values should you check before you administer her next dose?

    a. HCT and hemoglobin

    *b. BUN and creatinine

    c. SGOT and SGPT

    d. urine culture and sensitivity

6. Early symptoms of a hypersensitivity reaction to antitubercular drugs include

    a. nausea and diarrhea

    b. bradycardia and hypertension

    *c. fever and tachycardia

    d. bleeding gums

7. Your client, who weights 200 pounds, is to receive 1500 mg ethambutol daily. If the recommended dose is 15/mg/kg/ day, this dose is

    a. low

    *b. high

    c. appropriate

8. You should begin to see the therapeutic effects of antitubercular drug therapy in

    a. 5–7 days

    b. 7–10 days

    *c. 2–3 weeks

    d. 6 weeks

9. You will know that your client with tuberculosis is improving as the result of drug therapy when his

    a. weight decreases

    b. tidal volume increases

    *c. sputum decreases

    d. skin test improves

10. The recommended length of initial treatment for someone who has been exposed but has a negative tuberculin test is
    a. 10 days
    b. 3 months
    *c. 6 months
    d. 12 months

CHAPTER 39

1. Adverse effects of ganciclovir (Cytovene) that the nurse needs to assess for include
   a. stomatitis
   b. hypertension
   c. arrhythmias
   *d. thrombocytopenia

2. Mr. J. has herpes simplex encephalitis. An expected outcome after the administration of vidarabine (Vira-A) is
   *a. decreased fever
   b. decreased heart rate
   c. increased blood pressure
   d. increased respiratory rate

3. Live, attenuated viral vaccines should not be administered to persons who are
   a. diabetic
   *b. pregnant
   c. under age 2
   d. over age 70

4. Mr. J. is ordered vidarabine (Vira-A). The following statement by the client leads you to believe that he understands the teaching that you have done:
   a. "After I take this medication, I may notice tearing and nasal congestion."
   b. "After I administer the medication, I will apply cold compresses to my ears."
   c. "I should use this drug for no longer than 6 weeks."
   *d. "I may experience pain, itching, and inflammation of my eyelids."

5. Mr. J, a 21-year-old male, is being started on zidovudine (AZT) for treatment of AIDS. Which of the following statements by Mr. J. leads you to believe that he understands the teaching that you have done?
   a. "Zidovudine (AZT) inactivates the virus and prevents recurrence of the disease."
   b. "Zidovudine (AZT) therapy may result in the development of zidovudine–resistant viral strains."
   *c. "Zidovudine (AZT) slows the progression of the disease but does not cure it."
   d. "Zidovudine (AZT) prevents the occurrence of opportunistic infections."

6. Infants who are being treated with ribavirin (Virazole) for RSV should be assessed for
   a. hepatotoxicity
   b. renal failure
   c. ventricular tachycardia
   *d. deteriorating pulmonary function

7. Which of the following instructions should you give to Mrs. B, who is taking medication for a viral eye infection?
   a. "Use sterile gloves when you are applying the medication."
   *b. "Initially, you should administer the drops every 2–4 hours while you are awake."
   c. "The medication may temporarily cause yellowing of the sclera."
   d. "You should rinse your eye with sterile saline before applying the medication."

8. The use of amantadine (Symmetrel) for treatment of influenza A is recommended for use in
   a. all adults
   b. persons with a family history of heart disease
   *c. persons with chronic lung disease
   d. children under the age of 2

9. You are to administer acyclovir (Zovirax) intravenously. The recommended dose is 5 mg/kg q8h. Your client weighs 132 pounds. How much medication will you administer per dose?
   a. 100 mg
   b. 200 mg
   *c. 300 mg
   d. 400 mg

10. The following medications, if administered concurrently with zidovudine (AZT), will alter its effects:

    a. anticholinergics
    b. cholinergics
    c. corticosteroids
    *d. antineoplastics

CHAPTER 40

1. The drug most commonly used to treat infections caused by *Candida albicans* is

    a. acrisorcin (Akrinol)
    b. naftate (Tinactin)
    c. griseofulvin (Fulvicin)
    *d. nystatin (Mycostatin)

2. The following medication, if administered concurrently with ketoconazole (Nizoral), will decrease its effect:

    a. diuretics
    b. steroids
    *c. antacids
    d. antibiotics

3. Mrs. G., who weighs 90 pounds, is to receive griseofulvin (Fulvicin) 10 mg/kg daily. If Mrs. G. receives four doses daily, how much medication will she receive per dose?

    a. 75 mg
    *b. 100 mg
    c. 125 mg
    d. 150 mg

4. The following medications may be administered concurrently with amphotericin B (Fungizone) to try and minimize the adverse reactions to this medication:

    a. analgesics
    *b. antipyretics and antiemetics
    c. beta-adrenergic blockers
    d. steroids and diuretics

5. Mr. J. is receiving intravenous miconazole (Monistat). He should be observed for

    *a. anemia
    b. elevated BUN
    c. confusion
    d. diarrhea

6. The following statement by Mr. B. leads you to believe that he has understood the teaching that you have done regarding amphotericin B (Fungizone), "I could develop

    a. diabetes."
    b. liver necrosis."
    *c. renal damage."
    c. pancreatitis."

7. The following medication, if administered concurrently with griseofulvin (Fulvicin), will alter its effects:

    *a. gentamicin (Garamycin)
    b. furosemide (Lasix)
    c. prednisone (Deltasone)
    d. digoxin (Lanoxin)

8. Nystatin (Mycostatin) is ordered as a "swish." The client should be instructed to

    *a. rinse her mouth with the medication, then swallow it
    b. rinse her mouth, then spit the medication out
    c. swallow the medication, following it with 8 ounces of water
    d. dilute the medication and gargle with it

9. The following may be effective in treating tinea pedis

    a. acrisorcin (Akrinol)
    b. flucytosine (Ancobon)
    c. natamycin (Natacyn)
    *d. zinc undecylenate (Desenex)

10. You should give your client the following instructions regarding the administration of clotrimazole (Lotrimin):

    *a. fill the applicator with the medication and insert it into the vagina at bedtime
    b. apply the medication to the perineal area twice a day
    c. place the solution in a sitz bath and soak in it twice daily
    d. fill the applicator with the medication and insert into the vagina q4h and apply a sterile pad afterward

CHAPTER 41

1. During treatment of amebiasis with chloroquine (Aralen) you should be assessing the client for
   *a. diarrhea
   b. weight gain
   c. hypertension
   d. seizures

2. Persons using gamma benzene hexachloride (Kwell) should be instructed to report which of the following signs/symptoms to their physician?
   a. fatigue, cough, or dizziness
   *b. irritation, rash, or inflammation
   c. headache, nausea, or diarrhea
   d. anorexia, nausea, or vomiting

3. The following instructions should be given to a person who is starting on gamma benzene hexachloride (Kwell) for scabies:
   *a. bathe; apply lotion to all body surfaces except head and neck; leave on for 12–24 hours and bathe again
   b. apply lotion three times a day for a week
   c. take a warm shower in the morning; apply lotion all over your body and repeat before you go to bed
   d. wear gloves when applying the lotion to your body and keep it away from your eyes

4. For which of the following diagnoses should thiabendazole (Mintezol) be used with caution?
   a. hypothyroidism
   b. hypertension
   *c. renal insufficiency
   d. diabetes mellitus

5. The following statement by your client leads you to believe that she has understood the teaching that you have done regarding metronidazole (Flagyl):
   a. "I will refrain from operating heavy machinery while I am taking this medication."
   b. "I will avoid foods high in vitamin C."
   *c. "I will not drink alcohol while I am taking this medication."
   d. "I will contact my physician if I have diarrhea."

6. The following food, if taken with chloroquine phosphate (Aralen), may alter its effects:
   *a. citrus fruits
   b. red meats
   c. whole-grain wheat products
   d. dark-green leafy vegetables

7. Mr. B. is being treated for *Pneumocystis carinii* pneumonia with pentamidine isethionate (NebuPent). The following will be performed to assess the client for adverse effects of the medication:
   *a. CBC
   b. serum potassium
   c. daily blood pressure
   d. daily weight

8. Mr. B. is receiving quinine for malaria. He should be observed for cinchonism, symptoms of which include
   a. nausea, vomiting, and diarrhea
   *b. headache, tinnitus, and blurred vision
   c. chest pain, dyspnea, and tachycardia
   d. weakness, anorexia, and paresthesia

9. Chloroquine (Aralen) should be administered
   a. on an empty stomach
   b. with 8 ounces of water
   *c. with meals
   d. with orange juice followed by 8 ounces of water

10. Mrs. C., who is being treated with metronidazole (Flagyl) for giardiasis, calls to tell you there is blood in her feces. What is the best response to Mrs. C.?
    *a. "Come in immediately and we will do a stool specimen."
    b. "Don't be alarmed. We expect that your feces will change colors."
    c. "Make sure that you eat foods high in roughage and this will pass."
    d. "Flagyl is a dye that colors the feces bright red. Is that the color of your feces?"

CHAPTER 42

1. Passive nonspecific immunity
   *a. occurs when antibodies are formed by the immune system of another person and transferred to the host
   b. develops within 6 months after birth
   c. occurs when foreign substances stimulate production of antibodies
   d. develops when antibodies, which are innate to the organism, are stimulated to produce WBCs

2. Lymphokines
   *a. stimulate the growth of immune cells
   b. suppress T cell production
   c. inhibit protein production
   d. stimulate production of antibodies

3. A generalized response to cellular injury is
   a. decreased pH
   b. increased protein catabolism
   c. inhibition of cell growth
   *d. inflammation

4. Cytotoxic T cells
   a. secrete a toxic substance that kills the antigens
   b. bind to antigens and damage their cell membrane
   *c. inject fluid into the antigen cell, causing edema and death
   d. decreased the activities of the B cells

5. The following immunoglobulin is located in the tissues and is thought to be responsible for allergic reactions:
   a. IgG
   b. IgA
   c. IgM
   *d. IgE

6. Protein growth factors, secreted by WBCs, that regulate tissue inflammation and repair immune responses are
   a. interferons
   b. interleukins
   *c. cytokines
   d. monocytes

7. Interferons
   a. stimulate B lymphocyte activity
   b. interfere with multiplication of stem cells
   c. stimulate growth and differentiation of lymphoid cells into lymphocytes
   *d. interfere with the ability of viruses in infected cells to replicate

8. The levels of which of the following immunoglobulins are higher at birth than at 6 months of age?
   *a. IgG
   b. IgA
   c. IgM
   d. IgD

9. The following has the greatest impact on the immune system:
   a. sodium deficiency
   b. potassium excess
   c. magnesium excess
   *d. zinc deficiency

10. Administering immunizations
   a. strengthens antigens
   b. suppresses the normal response to antigens
   *c. helps clients develop a tolerance to certain substances
   d. decreases the numbers of T lymphocytes

CHAPTER 43

1. Administration of vaccines and toxoids is generally contraindicated in persons who
   a. have renal impairment
   b. have hepatic failure
   *c. are receiving steroids
   d. are over 65

2. Before administering a DTP vaccine, you should check the client's
   *a. temperature
   b. pulse
   c. blood pressure
   d. respiration

3. You should instruct the parents of a child receiving an immunization that it is common for children to experience
   a. nausea, vomiting, and diarrhea
   b. rash and swelling
   c. weakness and difficulty in walking
   *d. tenderness and redness at the site

4. Persons who have been immunized can develop serum sickness
   a. within minutes after the injection
   b. 12 hours after the injection
   *c. days or weeks after the injection
   d. 2–3 months after the injection

5. MMR (measles, mumps, and rubella) is administered initially at
   a. 1–2 months of age
   b. 3–4 months of age
   c. 5–6 months of age
   *d. 12–15 months of age

6. Tetanus toxoid should be administered to adults every
   a. year
   *b. 10 years
   c. 2 years
   d. 5 years

7. All of the following immunizations are routinely administered to American children except
   a. rubella and mumps vaccine
   b. poliovirus vaccine
   c. diphtheria, pertussis, and tetanus vaccine
   *d. tuberculosis vaccine

8. Hepatitis B vaccine is recommended for
   a. children under the age of 15
   *b. all children and persons at risk for contracting the disease
   c. persons with diabetes mellitus or renal disease
   d. persons over the age of 65

9. A rare reaction resulting from the administration of poliovirus vaccine is
   a. myasthenia gravis
   b. convulsions
   c. Huntington's chorea
   *d. Guillain-Barré syndrome

10. Anaphylaxis is most likely to occur within how many minutes after an immunizing agent is injected?
    a. 1 minute
    b. 5 minutes
    *c. 30 minutes
    d. 90 minutes

CHAPTER 44

1. Mr. G. is undergoing a bone marrow transplant. The drug that will be most effective in stimulating the production of granulocytes and macrophages is
   a. Bacille Calmette-Guérin (BCG)
   b. epoetin alfa (Epogen)
   c. filgrastim
   *d. sargramostim

2. Which of the following is considered a toxic side effect of interleukin-2 (aldesleukin) and would necessitate discontinuation of the drug?
   a. BP of 150/90
   *b. repetitive seizures
   c. blood sugar 300 mg/dL
   d. confusion

3. Mr. G. has just had a bone marrow transplant. Which of the following nursing diagnoses would take priority?
   a. body image disturbance related to illness
   *b. potential for infection related to immunosuppression
   c. anxiety related to diagnosis of cancer
   d. activity intolerance related to fatigue

4. Immunostimulants are being administered to Mr. C. to increase his WBC to
   a. 2–5 mm^3.
   *b. 5–10 mm^3.
   c. 15–20 mm^3.
   d. 20–24 mm^3.

5. An expected outcome after the administration of epoetin alfa (Epogen) is
   a. decreased RBC count
   *b. increased RBC count
   c. increased WBC count
   d. decreased WBC count

6. One of the adverse effects of the anti-AIDS drug zidovudine (Retrovir) that the nurse needs to assess for is
   a. decreased WBC count
   b. increased WBC count
   *c. decreased RBC count
   d. increased RBC count

7. Which of the following statements by Mr. G., who has renal carcinoma, leads you to believe that he has understood the teaching that you have done regarding interleukin-2 (aldesleukin)?
   *a. "This drug will inhibit tumor growth."
   b. "This drug will prevent me from developing a viral infection."
   c. "This drug will decrease the number of T cells."
   d. "This drug can cause renal failure."

8. For which of the following individuals would the use of BCG for bladder cancer be contraindicated?
   a. A person with a history of heart disease
   b. A person with a history of diabetes mellitus
   c. A person with a history of pulmonary fibrosis
   *d. A person with a history of a renal transplant

9. For persons who are immunosuppressed, the following lifestyle changes will enhance their immune mechanisms:
   a. eliminate fats and sugar from diet
   b. increase vitamin C in diet
   *c. avoid usage of tobacco and alcohol
   d. exercise daily

10. An expected outcome after the administration of immunostimulants is
    a. RBC of 3,000 mm^3
    *b. decreased numbers or severity of infections
    c. increased life expectancy
    d. a WBC of 20,000 mm^3

CHAPTER 45

1. One adverse effect of excessive immunosuppression is the development of
   a. liver failure
   b. kidney failure
   c. Kaposi's sarcoma
   *d. serious infection

2. Which of the following statements by 8-year-old B. J. leads you to believe that she has a good understanding of how to take cyclosporine (Sandimmune)?
   a. "I will take cyclosporine (Sandimmune) on an empty stomach."
   b. "I will follow the cyclosporine (Sandimmune) with 8 ounces of water."
   *c. "I will rinse out the glass after I have taken the cyclosporine (Sandimmune) and drink the rinse solution."
   d. "I will only take the medication after meals."

3. Persons receiving azathioprine (Imuran) should be observed for
   a. respiratory distress
   b. depression
   *c. abnormal bleeding
   d. severe diarrhea

4. Mr. J., who is receiving antithymocyte globulin (ATG; Atgam), experiences chest pain and difficulty breathing. Your initial nursing action should be
   *a. stop the drug infusion
   b. slow down the drug infusion
   c. contact the physician
   d. administer oxygen and nitroglycerin

5. Which of the following medications if administered concurrently with cyclosporine will decrease its effect?
   a. verapamil (Calan)
   *b. phenytoin (Dilantin)
   c. cimetidine (Tagamet)
   d. gentamicin

6. Which of the following instructions should be given to Mr. H., who is receiving methotrexate (Rheumatrex), to help him avoid the adverse effects of the medication?
   a. increase the fiber in your diet
   b. walk at least a mile every day and get a good night's sleep
   *c. drink at least 8 glasses of water daily
   d. wear protective clothing and use sunscreen to decrease your exposure to the sun

7. A nursing diagnosis that the nurse needs to include in his or her care plan after a renal transplant has been performed is

*a. social isolation

b. impaired gas exchange

c. impaired cardiac output

d. activity intolerance

8. Mr. P. is receiving immunosuppressive agents after a heart transplant. For which one of the following assessments would you contact the physician?

a. weight loss of 3 pounds

b. temperature of 36.8° C

*c. productive cough

d. hypoactive bowel sounds

9. After his liver transplant, Mr. J. receives immunosuppressants to prevent the following complication:

a. ascites

b. septicemia

*c. organ rejection

d. clotting off of graft

10. Persons receiving immunosuppressants after a kidney transplant should be observed for deterioration in kidney function. Which of the following lab studies would give you the earliest indication of a change in renal status?

a. BUN

b. serum sodium

c. serum potassium

*d. creatinine clearance

CHAPTER 46

1. The following causes an increased respiratory rate

*a. increased pCO_2

b. decreased pCO_2

c. increased O_2

d. decreased pH

2. The following disease process has the most significant impact on decreasing the compliance of the lungs:

*a. pulmonary fibrosis

b. pneumonia

c. anemia

d. cerebellar injury

3. The percentage of oxygen in room air is

*a. 21%

b. 28%

c. 35%

d. 40%

4. Air exchange takes place at the

a. trachea

b. bronchioles

*c. alveoli

d. all of the above

5. The following disease process has an impact on pulmonary perfusion:

a. hypertension

*b. anemia

c. cerebrovascular accident

d. pneumonia.

6. You would document the breathing pattern of a person with a respiratory rate of 12 as

a. normopnea.

b. tachypnea

*c. bradypnea

d. apnea

7. Mr. J. takes in 500 mL of air with each breath. This is referred to as

a. total lung capacity

b. residual volume

c. vital capacity

*d. tidal volume

8. The following regulates the rate and depth of respiration:

a. cerebrum

b. cerebellum

*c. medulla oblongata

d. reticular activating system

9. The following is responsible for bronchodilation:

a. parasympathetic nervous system

*b. sympathetic nervous system

c. medulla oblongata

d. cerebrum

10. Permanent damage can occur when the brain is deprived of oxygen for
    a. 1 minute
    b. 2 minutes
    c. 3 minutes
    *d. 4 minutes

CHAPTER 47

1. The following statement by a client using a beclomethasone (Vanceril) inhaler indicates adequate understanding of its use:
    a. "Because it is habit-forming, I will only use it once a day."
    *b. "If I need to use the drug more often than prescribed, I will call my doctor."
    c. "Nausea and vomiting are common with this drug."
    d. "I will keep the inhaler in a dry, warm place when it is not in use."

2. A newly diagnosed asthmatic should be instructed to avoid which of the following, which may cause her to experience bronchoconstriction?
    a. becoming fatigued
    b. direct sunlight
    *c. extremely cold temperatures
    d. food high in sodium

3. A dosage of theophylline may need to be increased if a client
    a. uses insulin
    b. takes cimetidine (Tagamet)
    c. exercises strenuously
    *d. smokes cigarettes

4. Mr. B. started on theophylline. You know that your teaching has been successful if he states, "I will
    *a. avoid caffeine."
    b. eat foods high in potassium."
    c. limit my fluid intake to 1000 mL a day."
    d. take the medicine on an empty stomach."

5. A client started on albuterol (Proventil) should be instructed that she may experience
    a. polydipsia
    *b. tachycardia
    c. hypotension
    d. diarrhea

6. The following statement indicates that your client has a good understanding of the teaching that you have done regarding inhalers:
    a. "I should hold my breath when administering a puff."
    *b. "The aerosol canister should be shaken well before using."
    c. "I need to take three short quick breaths when I administer the inhaler."
    d. "A second aerosol medication cannot be administered until 30 minutes after the first aerosol medication."

7. The following drug is effective in treating acute bronchospasm:
    a. ipratropium bromide (Atrovent)
    *b. epinephrine (Adrenalin)
    c. cromolyn (Intal)
    d. ephedrine

8. A client with chronic bronchitis is experiencing symptoms of respiratory distress. Which of the following symptoms indicate hypoxia?
    a. excessive mucus production
    b. expiratory wheezes and cyanosis
    c. activity intolerance
    *d. increased pulse

9. To avoid bronchospasm, the person who experiences acute asthma attacks should be advised to
    *a. use a bronchodilator inhaler prior to exercise
    b. avoid all strenuous exercise
    c. avoid all stressful situation
    d. limit time outdoors to 2 hours a day

10. All the following are helpful in removing secretions from the respiratory tract except
    a. drinking 2000 mL daily
    b. postural drainage
    c. deep breathing
    *d. administering of corticosteroids

11. A drug that decreases the effectiveness of bronchodilators is
    a. lithium (Eskalith)
    b. phenobarbital (Luminal)
    *c. propranolol (Inderal)
    d. cimetidine (Tagamet)

12. A client started on beclomethasone (Vanceril) may need additional teaching if he states the following: "I will . . .
    a. increase my intake of fluids."
    b. shake the aerosol canister well before using it."
    *c. not administer a second aerosol medication until an hour after taking this medication."
    d. rinse my mouth and the mouthpiece after each use."

13. The following statement made by your client leads you to believe that she has understood the teaching that you have done regarding cromolyn (Intal)
    a. "If I have an acute attack I will use the inhaler immediately."
    b. "I will cough after using this medication."
    c. "I will use a nasal decongestant along with this medication to enhance its effects."
    *d. "I will use this inhaler prior to exercise to prevent an asthma attack."

14. An expected outcome after the administration of aerosol bronchodilator is decreased dyspnea within
    *a. 1–2 minutes
    b. 3–5 minutes
    c. 10–15 minutes
    d. 20–30 minutes

15. When administering sympathomimetic bronchodilators, you can expect the client to experience
    *a. tachycardia
    b. sedation
    c. hypotension
    d. dry mouth

16. Corticosteroids are administered to clients in respiratory distress to
    a. depress the CNS
    b. reduce the respiratory rate
    c. produce bronchodilation
    *d. reduce airway inflammation

17. Bronchodilators may be used to treat the symptoms of hypoxia which include
    a. copious secretions
    b. diminished breath sounds

*c. anxiety and tachycardia
d. hypotension

18. Adrenergic bronchodilators should be used cautiously for clients with
    a. liver failure
    b. renal failure
    c. respiratory failure
    *d. heart failure

19. Ipratropium bromide (Atrovent) is used for
    *a. chronic bronchitis and emphysema
    b. mild to moderate asthma
    c. nasal congestion and throat irritation
    d. respiratory failure

20. The following indicates that the client is obtaining maximum benefit from the inhaler.
    a. He inhales as soon as the inhaler enters his mouth.
    *b. He holds his breath for several seconds after releasing the medication.
    c. He administers 3 doses of medication within a one-minute time frame.
    d. He exhales as soon as he compresses the inhaler.

CHAPTER 48

1. The following statement by your client indicates successful teaching concerning diphenhydramine hydrochloride (Benadryl):
    a. "I can still have my after-dinner drink."
    b. "I will eat a diet high in roughage while I am taking this medication."
    *c. "I should not operate heavy machinery when taking this medicine."
    d. "I can take this medication as frequently as I need it."

2. Antihistamines should be used with caution in individuals who have
    a. Parkinson's disease
    b. hypertension
    c. diabetes mellitus
    *d. prostatic hypertrophy

3. The following condition in your client's history could contraindicate the use of phenothiazines:

   a. Crohn's disease

   b. mitral valve prolapse

   *c. depression

   d. thyroid disease

4. Persons taking brompheniramine maleate (Dimetane) should be given the following instructions:

   a. do not drink more than 1500 mL daily

   b. only take the medication at bedtime

   c. eat foods high in vitamin C while you are taking this medication

   *d. avoid the use of alcohol while you are using this medication

5. The physician ordered meclizine hydrochloride (Antivert) for Mrs. B., who has Ménière's disease. Common adverse effects of this medication include

   a. dizziness and headache

   b. urinary retention and constipation

   *c. dry mouth and blurred vision

   d. diarrhea and abdominal cramping

6. When diphenhydramine hydrochloride (Benadryl) is administered parenterally, the nurse needs to observe the client for changes in

   a. heart rate

   *b. blood pressure

   c. respiratory rate

   d. orientation

7. The following antihistamine may also be effective as an antiemetic:

   a. loratidine (Claritin)

   b. clemastine fumarate (Tavist)

   *c. diphenhydramine hydrochloride (Benadryl)

   d. trimeprazine tartrate (Temaril)

8. An antihistamine that produces significant sedation is

   a. hydroxyzine (Vistaril)

   b. cyproheptadine (Periactin)

   *c. promethazine hydrochloride (Phenergan)

   d. dimenhydramine (Dramamine)

9. An overdose of antihistamines can result in

   a. a myocardial infarction

   b. a hypertensive crisis

   c. liver failure

   *d. hallucinations and convulsions

10. The following are adverse effects of diphenhydramine hydrochloride (Benadryl) except:

    a. constipation

    b. urinary retention

    *c. tachycardia

    d. drowsiness

11. A newer antihistamine that does not cause drowsiness is

    a. hydroxyzine (Vistaril)

    b. promethazine hydrochloride (Phenergan)

    c. dimenhydrinate (Dramamine)

    *d. loratidine (Claritin)

CHAPTER 49

1. A 14-year-old client receives acetylcysteine (Mucomyst) for which of the following conditions?

   a. severe cough

   b. pulmonary edema associated with heart failure

   *c. cystic fibrosis

   d. respiratory congestion related to chronic asthma

2. A female client has bronchitis, so the physician orders guaifenesin (Robitussin). The following instructions should be given:

   a. avoid becoming pregnant during guaifenesin therapy

   *b. avoid taking alcohol concurrently with this medication

   c. restrict fluids to 300 mL per day

   d. take the medication on an empty stomach

3. Acetylcysteine (Mucomyst)

   *a. decreases the viscosity of mucous secretions

   b. stimulates the bronchial cells to secrete watery mucous

   c. stimulates ciliary activity

   d. increases the tenaciousness of bronchial

secretions

4. The following statements by a client who is to take an antitussive with codeine indicates that your teaching has been effective:

    a. "I will take this medication anytime I start to cough."

    b. "This medication may make me anxious and nervous."

    c. "I should call the physician if I develop nausea, diarrhea, or stomach cramps while taking this medication."

    *d. "This medication can cause drowsiness, so I will avoid driving while I use it."

5. The following is a common complaint from a client receiving acetylcysteine (Mucomyst) by nebulizer treatment:

    a. "This medication gives me palpitations."

    b. "I lose my ability to cough after taking the treatment."

    *c. "The mist I breathe in smells and tastes awful."

    d. "I get a headache every time I have a treatment."

6. The following statement by your client leads you to believe that he needs additional instruction regarding his nasal decongestant:

    a. "I will blow my nose before instilling the nasal spray."

    b. "I will report any dizziness, drowsiness, or rapid pulse."

    c. "I will drink 2000–3000 mL of fluid daily."

    *d. "I will use it only when I have nasal discharge."

7. An adverse reaction commonly experienced by persons taking nasal decongestants is

    a. diarrhea

    *b. dry mouth

    c. rash

    d. headache

8. The following medications, if administered with dextromethorphan, could cause apnea:

    a. calcium channel blockers

    *b. MAO inhibitors

    c. beta blockers

    d. thiazide diuretics

9. The following medications, if administered with nasal decongestants, increase the risk of cardiac arrhythmias:

    a. atropine

    b. propranolol (Inderal)

    *c. theophylline

    d. furosemide (Lasix)

10. The following instructions should be given to the mother of a 3-month-old infant who has an upper respiratory tract infection and has been placed on nasal decongestants:

    *a. instill the medication 20–30 minutes before feeding

    b. keep the baby on clear liquids until the nasal discharge has resolved

    c. start the baby on cereal because she is having difficulty sucking right now

    d. give the medication immediately before feeding, followed by 4 ounces of water

11. Persons taking a narcotic antitussive need to be observed for

    *a. respiratory depression

    b. constipation

    c. tachycardia

    d. muscle rigidity

12. A client with cancer of the lung complains of a persistent cough that interrupts his sleep. Which of the following assessments should the nurse perform before contacting the physician to ask for an order for an antitussive?

    a. count the number and length of each coughing spell

    b. count his respiratory and pulse rate for a full minute

    c. determine pO_2 levels

    *d. observe for any sputum and evaluate its color and consistency

13. A client diagnosed with pneumonia is using acetylcysteine (Mucomyst). A nursing action that would be appropriate is

    a. discouraging resting during the day

    b. checking breath sounds every hour

    c. maintaining bedrest to avoid complications caused by Mucomyst

    *d. encouraging 2000–3000 mL fluid intake daily

14. Instructions you should give a client who is taking saturated solution of potassium iodine (SSKI) include

    a. always take this medication on an empty stomach

    *b. dilute the medication in a full glass of juice

    c. do not drink anything for an hour after this medication

    d. this medication should be taken 20–30 minutes before meals

CHAPTER 50

1. The valve that separates the left atrium and ventricle is the

    *a. mitral

    b. pulmonic

    c. aortic

    d. tricuspid

2. The ability of the heart to pump efficiently depends upon the client's

    a. age

    b. venous capacitance

    *c. heart rate

    d. blood pressure

3. The following area of the heart can beat independently with a rate of 30–40:

    a. the AV node

    b. the bundle of His

    c. the Purkinje fibers

    *d. the ventricle

4. Red blood cells are produced by the

    a. reticuloendothelial tissues

    b. lymphatic tissue

    *c. bone marrow

    d. liver

5. The blood does all of the following except

    a. help regulate body temperature

    b. transport oxygen

    c. protect the body from invading organisms

    *d. regulate metabolism of glucose

6. The middle layer of an artery is composed of

    *a. muscle and elastic tissue

    b. connective tissue

    c. fibrous tissue

    d. reticular tissue

7. Red blood cells are also referred to as

    a. leukocytes

    *b. erythrocytes

    c. thrombocytes

    d. monocytes

8. The fibrous sac enclosing the heart is the

    a. endocardium

    b. myocardium

    c. epicardium

    *d. pericardium

9. Vessels that carry large molecules of protein and fat are the

    a. arteries

    b. veins

    c. capillaries

    *d. lymphatic vessels

10. The component of the blood necessary for maintaining colloid osmotic pressure is

    *a. albumin

    b. fibrinogen

    c. gamma globulin

    d. platelets

CHAPTER 51

1. You should withhold digoxin (Lanoxin) and notify the physician if the client's

    a. respiratory rate falls below 14

    b. history reveals liver failure

    *c. pulse is 54 beats per minute

    d. blood pressure is 72/40 mm Hg

2. A medication that increases the force of the contractions of the heart has a

    a. positive chronotropic effect

    *b. positive inotropic effect

    c. negative inotropic effect

    d. negative dromotropic effect

3. The following diet is the most desirable for a client receiving cardiac glycosides:

    a. high-sodium, low-potassium, high-fat

    b. low-sodium, low-potassium, low-fat

    c. high-iron, high-calcium, high-potassium

    *d. low-sodium, high-potassium, low-fat

4. A client in the late stages of digoxin (Lanoxin) toxicity will exhibit

    *a. tachycardia

    b. anorexia, headache

    c. decreased urinary output

    d. bradycardia

5. A loading dose of digoxin (Lanoxin) is ordered. You would recognize that the physician ordered the correct dose if it was

    a. 0.25 mg IV q4h × 24 hrs

    *b. 0.25 mg PO q8h × 3 doses

    c. 0.25 mg PO qd

    d. 1 mg IM q12h × 24 hrs

6. A client has a serum digoxin level of 3.3 ng/mL. You should

    a. administer the next dose as scheduled

    b. assess the client's pulse and blood pressure before the next dose

    *c. withhold the next dose and contact the physician

    d. administer Digibind

7. Heart failure results in increased preload, which is the

    *a. amount of blood returning to the heart

    b. resistance the heart must overcome

    c. amount of blood pooled in the extremities

    d. pulse rate caused by venous distention

8. Your client is receiving digoxin (Lanoxin) and furosemide (Lasix). In the morning she complains of a headache and nausea. What will you do first?

    a. contact her physician immediately

    *b. check her lab values and vital signs

    c. administer Tylenol and Maalox

    d. give her clear liquids and have her lie down

9. A client, admitted with atrial fibrillation last evening, was given two doses of digoxin (Lanoxin) totaling 1 mg. His digoxin level this morning is 0.4 ng/mL. You know that this is

    *a. lower than a therapeutic level

    b. within a therapeutic range

    c. slightly higher than a therapeutic range

    d. a toxic level

10. The following statement by your client leads you to believe that she understands the teaching that you have done about digoxin. "I will

    a. take the medication in the morning before I get out of bed."

    *b. take my pulse every day."

    c. stop the medicine if my pulse is below 60."

    d. eat foods high in potassium."

11. When administering amrinone (Inocor), you should observe the client for the following adverse effect:

    a. hypoglycemia

    b. confusion

    *c. hypotension

    d. seizures

12. Cardiac glycosides are used to

    a. decrease cardiac output

    b. decrease afterload

    c. increase ventricular rate

    *d. increase the force of the contraction of the heart

13. The following is an outcome associated with the administration of digoxin:

    a. increased heart size

    *b. increased urinary output

    c. decreased respiratory rate

    d. increased blood sugar

14. Persons taking digoxin (Lanoxin) and phenytoin (Dilantin) concurrently may have

    a. decreased Dilantin levels

    b. elevated digoxin levels

    *c. decreased digoxin levels

    d. elevated Dilantin levels

15. The following medication, when administered concurrently with digoxin, will increase the serum digoxin concentration:
    a. nitroglycerin (Nitro-Bid)
    b. furosemide (Lasix)
    c. glyburide (DiaBeta)
    *d. verapamil (Calan)

16. The following electrolyte imbalance can precipitate digoxin toxicity:
    a. hyperkalemia
    *b. hypokalemia
    c. hypernatremia
    d. hyponatremia

17. The following should be assessed while your client is receiving enalapril (Vasotec) for heart failure:
    a. respiratory status
    b. liver function
    *c. potassium levels
    d. blood glucose levels

CHAPTER 52

1. The following would be an adverse effect of quinidine therapy:
    a. seizures
    b. rash
    c. headache
    *d. diarrhea

2. The following behavior by persons receiving propranolol (Inderal) indicates that your teaching has been successful. They
    a. increase their fluid intake to 3000 cc/day
    *b. report a weight gain of over 2 pounds in 1 week
    c. take multivitamins daily
    d. take their pulse once a week

3. Side effects of lidocaine (Xylocaine) therapy that the nurse should be observing for include
    a. dysphagia
    *b. disorientation
    c. excessive bruising
    d. tinnitus

4. After you have administered a bolus of lidocaine, you will run a continuous infusion at the following rate:
    a. 0.25–0.75 mg/min
    b. 10–20 mg/min
    *c. 1–4 mg/min
    d. 6–8 mg/min

5. The following drug may be used to terminate supraventricular tachycardia:
    a. lidocaine (Xylocaine)
    b. flecainide (Tambocor)
    *c. adenosine (Adenocard)
    d. bretylium (Bretylol)

6. Persons taking a beta-adrenergic blocker such as propranolol (Inderal) for its antiarrhythmic effect should be observed for
    a. tachycardia
    b. hypertension
    *c. heart failure
    d. diarrhea

7. The cardiac antiarrhythmic that can cause gingival hyperplasia is
    *a. phenytoin (Dilantin)
    b. propranolol (Inderal)
    c. lidocaine (Xylocaine)
    d. esmolol (Brevibloc)

8. Mr. J. is being sent home on disopyramide (Norpace) for atrial fibrillation. He asks you why he must continue to take this drug. Your best response would be, "Atrial fibrillation
    *a. can lead to the formation of clots in the heart."
    b. will result in the ventricles beating independently."
    c. may result in death."
    d. can cause edema in your extremities."

9. The physician plans on treating your client's atrial fibrillation with digoxin (Lanoxin). Prior to initiating treatment, your client should be taught to
    *a. check her pulse daily
    b. check her blood pressure daily
    c. contact her physician if her urinary output increases
    d. monitor her weight and blood sugar daily

10. The following statement by your client leads you to believe that she has a good understanding of the teaching that you have done regarding quinidine. "I will
    a. take the medication with citrus juice."
    b. increase the fiber in my diet."
    *c. take the medication with meals."
    d. limit my salt intake."

11. A factor that would necessitate that the dosage of disopyramide (Norpace) be reduced would be
    a. immobility
    b. hypertension
    *c. renal impairment
    d. chronic diarrhea

CHAPTER 53

1. A client is admitted with uncontrolled chest pain. He is currently taking nitroglycerin (Nitro-Bid). His physician orders nifedipine (Procardia) added to his regimen. You should observe the client for
    a. hypokalemia
    b. renal insufficiency
    *c. hypotension
    d. bradycardia

2. The following condition may preclude the use of beta-adrenergic blockers:
    a. migraine headache
    b. hypertension
    *c. heart failure
    d. tachycardia

3. The following statement by your client would indicate an understanding of how to take sublingual nitroglycerin:
    a. "Once I get a headache I know that a therapeutic level has been reached and I will take no more medication."
    *b. "I can take up to 3 tablets at 5 minute intervals."
    c. "I can take as much nitroglycerin as I need because it is not habit forming."
    d. "If I become dizzy after taking the medication, I should stop taking it."

4. Beta-adrenergic blockers help to control angina but can cause
    a. increased heart rate
    b. increased oxygen consumption
    *c. decreased contraction of the heart
    d. decreased urinary output

5. Your client can expect relief of chest pain when she takes nitroglycerin in
    *a. 1–3 minutes
    b. 5–10 minutes
    c. 15–20 minutes
    d. 30–60 minutes

6. When instructing your client about a nitroglycerin patch, you should tell him that the advantage of the patch is that it
    a. only has to be administered once a week
    b. is more effective than tablets in treating angina
    *c. has a longer duration of action
    d. is faster acting than the tablets

7. Which statement by your client would lead you to believe that he has understood the teaching that you have done regarding angina?
    a. "I will not exercise because it precipitates angina."
    b. "As long as I take the medicine, I need to make no lifestyle change."
    c. "There is no correlation between my hypertension and angina."
    *d. "Heavy meals and cigarette smoking can precipitate an anginal attack."

8. Persons taking calcium channel blockers can experience
    a. hypertension and tachycardia
    *b. headache and dizziness
    c. flushing and rash
    d. nausea and diarrhea

9. Persons receiving nifedipine (Procardia) should be assessed for
    a. ascites
    b. asthma
    *c. peripheral edema
    d. tetany

CHAPTER 54

1. Vasopressor drugs are useful in treating
   a. postural hypotension
   *b. hypotension resulting from decreased cardiac output
   c. hypotension secondary to anemia
   d. hypotension secondary to anesthesia

2. A client is admitted to the ICU with a diagnosis of cardiogenic shock. Which one of the following should be reported to the physician?
   a. temperature of 100.8° F
   b. nausea and vomiting
   *c. urinary output of less than 30 cc/hr
   d. abdominal distention

3. The following nursing diagnoses would be a priority for a client with hypovolemic shock:
   *a. altered tissue perfusion
   b. activity intolerance
   c. social isolation
   d. altered bowel elimination

4. The following nursing actions would take priority for a person with hypovolemic shock related to blood loss:
   a. monitor intake and weight
   b. assess lung and bowel sounds
   c. check peripheral pulses and skin temp
   *d. check blood pressure and pulse

5. A client in your unit has a gunshot wound. His family is very concerned about him and questions why the dobutamine (Dobutrex) is being used. Your best reply is
   a. " We are giving this drug to increase Mr. G.'s heart rate and blood pressure."
   b. "This drug will improve Mr. G.'s condition."
   *c. "This drug will increase the force of contraction of his heart and increase the blood supply to his vital organs."
   d. "We want to slow down Mr. G.'s heart rate and increase his blood pressure, and this drug will do that."

6. Mr. J. is started on an IV drip of dopamine (Intropin) for hypotension after open heart surgery. Identify which of these adverse effects you will be assessing for:
   a. hypertension
   *b. tachycardia
   c. bradycardia
   d. cyanosis

7. Mr. P. is being treated for hypotension with dopamine (Intropin) and begins to complain of chest pain. Which of the following antianginal drugs would you question if they were ordered?
   a. nitroglycerin (Nitro-Bid)
   *b. propranolol (Inderal)
   c. diltiazem (Cardizem)
   d. amyl nitrite

8. An IV of 200 mg of dopamine (Intropin) in 250 cc of D5W (800 µg/1 cc) is ordered. If the physician wants the client to receive 400 µg/minute, how fast will you run the IV? (Use micro-drip tubing 1 cc = 60 gtts.)
   a. 15 gtts.
   *b. 30 gtts.
   c. 60 gtts.
   d. 90 gtts.

9. If you note that levarterenol (Levophed) has extravasated, you should
   a. administer a beta-adrenergic blocker
   b. apply a tourniquet
   c. apply ice and elevate the extremity
   *d. administer phentolamine (Regitine) at the site

10. The following statement by a client leads you to believe he has understood the teaching you had done regarding dobutamine (Dobutrex):
   a. "If I continue to have problems once I leave this unit, I can take dobutamine (Dobutrex) orally."
   *b. "They will be monitoring my pulse, blood pressure, and urinary output frequently."
   c. "I can expect severe headaches and I will not worry."
   d. "Nausea and vomiting are common, so I will stick to clear liquids."

11. The major advantage of dobutamine (Dobutrex) over dopamine (Intropin) for clients in cardiogenic shock is
   a. it produces less hypotension as a side effect
   b. acute renal failure is rarely seen with this medication

*c. it does not produce systemic vasoconstriction

d. the dosage of the medication is much smaller

CHAPTER 55

1. When assessing a client, the following disorder from a client's history would be a contraindication for the use of calcium channel blockers:

   *a. heart failure

   b. severe hypertension

   c. increased intracranial pressure

   d. asthma

2. A client is receiving captopril (Capoten). Identify which of the following problems it might be used to treat:

   *a. chronic hypertension

   b. venous thrombosis

   c. hypertensive crisis

   d. unstable angina pectoris

3. A pregnant client admitted to the hospital with pregnancy-induced hypertension is ordered to receive hydralazine (Apresoline) 20 mg IV for a blood pressure greater than 190/100. The best response of the nurse to this order is to

   a. call the physician because the drug is inappropriate for a pregnant client

   *b. give the medication as ordered

   c. give half the dose first to see how it affects the blood pressure

   d. hold the medication and call the physician because the dose is too large

4. A client is started on trandolapril (Mavik). Instruct the client that a common adverse effect of ACE inhibitor therapy is

   a. sedation

   *b. persistent cough

   c. tachycardia

   d. rash

5. The physician prescribes captopril (Capoten) for your client. You know that your teaching has been effective if your client says, "I will

   a. limit my fluid intake to 1200 cc daily."

   *b. make sure that I rise slowly from a supine position."

   c. take a laxative along with the antihypertensive medication."

   d. decrease my intake of foods high in potassium."

6. The following represents the most important outcome for Mr. J., who has recently been diagnosed with hypertension:

   a. verbalization of an understanding of his medical regimen

   b. confirmation that his prescriptions have been filled

   *c. evidence of a diastolic BP below 90

   d. evidence of a pulse below 80

7. Your client, who is being treated for hypertension, should be instructed to avoid foods high in sodium, which include

   a. citrus fruits

   b. baked potatoes

   *c. sandwich meats

   d. red meat

8. The following statement by your client would indicate a good understanding of what you have taught her regarding hypertension:

   a. "If I think that my blood pressure is high, I will take an extra pill."

   b. "When I no longer have headaches, I can stop taking the medication."

   c. "For relaxation, I will soak in a hot tub."

   *d. "If I feel dizzy, I will still take my medication and have my blood pressure checked."

9. Your client is to be placed on reserpine (Serpasil). Prior to administration of this medication, you should ask if your client has a history of

   *a. depression

   b. glaucoma

   c. diabetes mellitus

   d. seizures

10. Besides decreasing Mr. P.'s blood pressure, an expected outcome after the administration of propranolol (Inderal) is

    a. increased urinary output

    *b. decreased heart rate

    c. increased respiratory rate

    d. decreased urinary output

11. Your client should be aware of the following side effects associated with hydralazine (Apresoline) therapy:

    *a. sodium and water retention

    b. potassium loss

    c. blood dyscrasias

    d. constipation

12. Persons experiencing both hypertension and angina are bested treated with

    *a. beta-adrenergic blockers

    b. direct-acting vasodilators

    c. thiazide diuretics

    d. ACE inhibitors

13. Angiotensin-converting enzyme (ACE) inhibitors work by

    a. stimulating the release of renin

    *b. blocking the enzyme that converts angiotensin I to angiotensin II

    c. increasing peripheral resistance

    d. blocking SNS impulses in the heart and brain

14. Your client, who is receiving propranolol (Inderal), has the following complaints. Which of the following may be directly related to the Inderal?

    a. headache

    b. chest pain

    c. palpitations

    *d. dizziness

CHAPTER 56

1. Diuretics and albumin are used together to treat edema that occurs because of

    a. decreased capillary permeability

    b. decreased capillary hydrostatic pressure

    *c. decreased plasma osmotic pressure

    d. decreased serum sodium levels

2. When loop diuretics are administered intravenously, you can expect to see a response to the medication in

    *a. 5 to 10 minutes

    b. 15 to 20 minutes

    c. 30 to 60 minutes

    d. 2 hours

3. Your client, an insulin-dependent diabetic, is to receive hydrochlorothiazide (HydroDIURIL). Prior to administering it, you should inform her that

    *a. her insulin dose may need to be increased

    b. her insulin dose may need to be decreased

    c. she will need to check her blood sugars four times a day

    d. she will need to have a creatinine clearance done once a month

4. When evaluating your client, who is receiving hydrochlorothiazide (HydroDIURIL), which of the following lab value deviations may be related to the medication?

    *a. elevated uric acid levels

    b. reduced BUN levels

    c. a serum potassium level of 5.5 mEq/liter

    d. a blood sugar of 66

5. The following statement by your client makes you believe that she understands your teaching about diuretics:

    *a. "I will weigh myself once a week and report significant changes."

    b. "I will no longer have to watch what I eat."

    c. "If my leg gets swollen again, I'll take an additional pill."

    d. "I will take my medication at night."

6. Mr. C. is admitted and the physician draws a serum potassium. Which of the following values is within the normal range?

    a. 2.1–3.4 mEq/liter

    *b. 3.5–5.0 mEq/liter

    c. 5.1–6.5 mEq/liter

    d. 6.6–7.9 mEq/liter

7. Mrs. B. is started on furosemide (Lasix) 40 mg daily. You will check her lab values on a regular basis because you know a side effect of this medication is

    a. hyperchloremia

    *b. hyponatremia

    c. hyperkalemia

    d. hypophosphatemia

8. When administering intravenous furosemide (Lasix), you will administer it slowly, because if it is administered rapidly, it can cause
   a. renal failure
   b. respiratory distress
   c. blindness
   *d. hearing loss

9. Spironolactone (Aldactone) should not be administered to persons with
   a. diabetes mellitus
   *b. elevated serum potassium levels
   c. elevated serum sodium levels
   d. hypertension

10. Which of the following is an osmotic diuretic?
    a. spironolactone (Aldactone)
    b. bumetanide (Bumex)
    *c. mannitol (Osmitrol)
    d. ethacrynic (Edecrin)

11. A client would receive furosemide (Lasix) for the following condition:
    a. hypotension
    b. myxedema
    *c. anasarca
    d. cerebral aneurysm

12. A client, in acute heart failure with severe respiratory distress, is to receive furosemide (Lasix) 100 mg IV. Lasix comes in 100 mg/10 mL. How will you administer the medication?
    *a. as rapidly as possible
    b. push it in over 3 minutes
    c. flush the line with normal saline, give 1 mL/min, flush when finished
    d. mix it in an IV piggyback and drop it in over 30 minutes

13. The following may be an indication that the nurse is giving IV push furosemide (Lasix) too rapidly:
    *a. the client has a sudden urge to void
    b. the client complains of blurred vision
    c. the client states that his ears are "plugged up"
    d. the client complains of nausea and vomits

14. A client receiving hydrochlorothiazide (HCTZ) for hypertension should be observed for the following adverse effect:
    a. tachycardia
    b. chronic diarrhea
    c. decreased chloride levels
    *d. elevated uric acid levels

15. A common side effect that a client receiving furosemide (Lasix) for hypertension could experience is
    a. rapid heart rate
    b. chronic fatigue
    *c. abdominal and leg cramps
    d. blurred vision

CHAPTER 57

1. A 19-year-old female, who takes birth control pills and is a heavy smoker, develops a thrombus in her leg. She is admitted to the hospital and is started on heparin. The following nursing actions would be the most important to this client:
   a. allow her to go the designated smoking area to prevent nicotine withdrawal
   b. give her Motrin for headaches and joint pain
   *c. maintain her on strict bed rest
   d. provide active ROM every 4 hours to prevent pneumonia and joint stiffness

2. A client receives IV heparin 5000 U qh. A partial thromboplastin time (PTT) is drawn a half an hour before the 8:00 a.m dose; the PTT is at 92 seconds. The most appropriate action would be to
   a. give the next two doses at the same time
   b. give the dose and chart the results
   c. check the client's vital signs and place him or her on bleeding precautions
   *d. hold the dose and call the result to the physician

3. A diabetic client is receiving tissue plasminogen activator (t-PA) for an acute myocardial infarction and has a blood sugar of 480. How will the 10 units of regular insulin be administered?
   a. subcutaneously
   b. placed in the IV bag
   *c. given IV push
   d. via inhalation

4. The effects of warfarin sodium (Coumadin) are monitored by the following lab test
   a. CBC
   b. APTT
   *c. INR
   d. BUN

5. Bleeding resulting from the administration of heparin is treated with
   a. vitamin E
   b. vitamin K
   *c. protamine sulfate
   d. calcium gluconate

6. You know that your client needs additional teaching regarding anticoagulants if he states, "I will
   a. carry a Medic Alert card with me."
   b. report to the lab once a month."
   *c. use aspirin for arthritis pain."
   d. use an electric razor."

7. Persons taking Coumadin should minimize foods high in vitamin K, including
   a. eggs
   b. dairy products
   c. citrus fruits
   *d. green leafy vegetables

8. You know that your teaching about Coumadin is successful if your client states
   a. "If I miss a dose, I will take two pills the next day."
   *b. "I will not drink alcoholic beverages."
   c. "I will increase the dark-green leafy vegetables in my diet."
   d. "I can still take over-the-counter medications if I have a cold."

9. A client receiving Coumadin has blood in his urinary drainage bag this morning. After reporting your observations to the physician, you will administer
   a. Amicar
   b. platelets
   c. protamine sulfate
   *d. vitamin K

10. Mr. L., who is receiving streptokinase for a myocardial infarction, passes a large amount of blood with his stool. After you notify the physician, you will expect to
    a. reduce the streptokinase and administer vitamin K
    b. stop the streptokinase and administer protamine sulfate
    c. reduce the streptokinase and administer heparin
    *d. stop the streptokinase and administer Amicar

11. Your client, admitted with thrombophlebitis, is being sent home on Lovenox. He has a good understanding of why Lovenox is being used if he states that it will
    *a. inhibit the formation of additional clots
    b. eliminate certain clotting factors
    c. prevent the blood from clotting
    d. dissolve the clot

12. When a client is a receiving a continuous drip of heparin 1000 units/hr, you should
    *a. avoid intramuscular injections
    b. assess for symptoms of respiratory depression
    c. take hourly urinary outputs
    d. take hourly vital signs

13. When you administer heparin, you should
    *a. apply pressure to the injection site
    b. insert the needle at a 45-degree angle
    c. gently massage the site after the injection
    d. use the Z-track method

CHAPTER 58

1. The following antilipemic is used for the treatment of types IV and V hyperlipidemia:
   a. colestipol
   b. fluvastatin (Lescol)
   *c. gemfibrozil (Lopid)
   d. lovastatin (Mevacor)

2. Adverse effects of antilipemics include
   *a. nausea, flatulence, and constipation
   b. abdominal cramping and distention
   c. anorexia and fatigue
   d. belching, hiccups, and dizziness

3. To minimize the flushing associated with nicotinic acid, the client should
   a. take the medication with meals
   *b. take ASA 30 minutes before the medication
   c. drink citrus juice with the medication
   d. take it at bedtime with milk

CHAPTER 59

1. An organ that regulates glucose metabolism and blood sugar levels is the
   a. liver
   b. gallbladder
   *c. pancreas
   d. small intestine

2. A substance required for digestion and absorption of fats and fat-soluble vitamins is
   a. hydrochloric acid
   *b. bile
   c. pancreatic juice
   d. gastric juice

3. When liver functioning is impaired, toxic levels of this substance can build up and result in coma or death:
   *a. ammonia
   b. hormones
   c. glucose
   d. bilirubin

4. This organ secretes the intrinsic factor that is necessary for the absorption of vitamin B:
   a. pancreas
   b. liver
   c. gallbladder
   *d. stomach

5. The bile duct empties into the
   *a. duodenum
   b. jejunum
   c. ileum
   d. cecum

6. In this portion of the intestine, water is absorbed:
   a. duodenum
   b. jejunum

   c. ileum
   *d. cecum

7. When mucous secretion is absent, the following will occur:
   a. diarrhea
   *b. ulceration
   c. constipation
   d. distention

8. Saliva has a pH of
   a. 2 to 3
   b. 4 to 5
   *c. 6 to 7
   d. 8 or above

9. Stimulation of the sympathetic nervous system will
   a. increase peristalsis
   *b. decrease peristalsis
   c. have no impact on peristalsis
   d. result in hyperactive bowel sounds

10. This hormone is released when fats are present in the duodenum:
    *a. enterogastrone
    b. gastrin
    c. pepsin
    d. lipase

CHAPTER 60

1. You should avoid rapid IV infusion of cimetidine (Tagamet) because it can cause
   a. hypothermia
   b. hypertension
   *c. confusion
   d. seizures

2. Side effects related to cimetidine therapy include
   a. bradycardia
   *b. abdominal pain and diarrhea
   c. visual disturbances
   d. macular rash and cough

3. Mr. S., who receives aluminum hydroxide (Amphojel) via nasogastric tube every 4 hours, should be observed for
   a. hypersensitivity reaction
   b. hypocalcemia
   c. metabolic alkalosis
   *d. constipation

4. The following is a contraindication for the use of metoclopramide (Reglan):
   a. anorexia
   b. depression
   *c. Parkinson's disease
   d. hypotension

5. When administering metoclopramide (Reglan), you should assess the client for the following adverse effects:
   a. photophobia
   b. bradycardia
   *c. restlessness
   d. excessive bruising

6. Your client, with peptic ulcer disease, is started on sucralfate (Carafate). A potential nursing diagnosis related to this medication is
   *a. alteration in bowel elimination: constipation
   b. potential for injury: bleeding
   c. impaired nutrition related to nausea
   d. electrolyte imbalance

7. For the best effectiveness, you should administer sucralfate at the following time:
   a. with meals
   b. with an antacid
   *c. 1 hour before meals
   d. after each meal

8. Your client will receive ranitidine (Zantac) 150 mg PO at bedtime. Prior to administration, you should inform the client that common side effects related to this medication are
   a. fever and chills
   *b. headache
   c. visual disturbances
   d. anxiety and depression

9. Ranitidine (Zantac) should be cautiously administered to individuals with evidence of
   *a. renal disease
   b. diabetes mellitus
   c. pulmonary disease
   d. migraine headaches

CHAPTER 61

1. Your client is to begin taking psyllium hydrophilic mucilloid (Metamucil) daily. You should include the following information in your discharge plan:
   *a. drink at least 8 ounces of fluid with the medication
   b. mix the medication with your food at your evening meal
   c. add all of the medications to the mucilloid
   d. discontinue the mucilloid if no bowel movement is noted in 24 hours

2. The followings drugs slow intestinal motility and put persons at risk for constipation:
   *a. tricyclic antidepressants
   b. thiazide diuretics
   c. calcium channel blockers
   d. thyroid preparations

3. A client who is taking a senna preparation (Senokot) calls you because she has noticed that her urine is a deep red and she thinks she is bleeding. Your best response would be
   a. "Come in immediately and we will take a urine specimen."
   b. "Go directly to the emergency room and the doctor will meet you there."
   *c. "The medication you are taking can color the urine different shades of red."
   d. "Drink 2000–3000 cc of acidic fluid every day and your urine will clear."

4. The following statement by your client leads you to believe that he has understood how to use bulk-forming laxatives:
   *a. "I will mix the medication with 4–8 ounces of liquid and follow it by an additional 4–8 ounces."
   b. "I will mix the dry medication with applesauce."
   c. "I will use milk of magnesia in conjunction with this medication until I am having daily bowel movements."

d. "I will decrease the roughage in my diet while I am using this medication."

5. An adverse effect of administration of stimulant cathartics is
    a. nausea
    b. vomiting
    *c. diarrhea
    d. lower GI bleeding

6. Long-term administration of mineral oil can decrease the absorption of
    a. vitamin B_{12}
    b. vitamin C
    *c. vitamin D
    d. vitamin B_2

7. Long-term use of saline cathartics can result in
    a. hypomagnesemia
    *b. hypernatremia
    c. hypochloremia
    d. hyperphosphatemia

8. Administering castor oil the following way would make it more palatable:
    a. heat it
    *b. chill it
    c. dilute it with water
    d. flavor it with peppermint

9. The safest and most effective way to treat constipation in children is with
    a. milk of magnesia
    b. sorbitol
    c. Dulcolax suppositories
    *d. glycerin suppositories

10. An alcoholic with chronic liver failure could use the following laxative to lower his serum ammonia levels:
    a. docusate sodium (Colace)
    b. polyethylene glyco-electrolyle solution (GoLYTELY).
    *c. lactulose (Chronulac)
    d. sorbitol

11. After surgery for a peptic ulcer, your client is receiving morphine sulfate 2 mg q4h, tetracycline 250 mg q6h, cimetidine (Tagamet) 300 mg q6h, and acetaminophen (Tylenol) 600 mg q4h. Which of the medications above is most likely to cause constipation?
    a. tetracycline
    b. cimetidine (Tagamet)
    *c. morphine sulfate
    d. acetaminophen (Tylenol)

CHAPTER 62

1. Psyllium hydrophilic mucilloid (Metamucil) should be avoided if Mrs. V. has
    a. arthritis
    b. glaucoma
    c. hypertension
    *d. diabetes mellitus

2. An expected outcome of the administration of psyllium hydrophilic mucilloid (Metamucil) is a regular bowel movement
    a. after 1 week
    *b. within 1 to 3 days
    c. after 2 weeks
    d. within 12 hours

3. Evidence of the following indicates that a client taking pancrelipase (Cotazym) needs to have his medication altered:
    *a. steatorrhea
    b. flatulence
    c. abdominal cramping
    d. excessive burping

4. A client receiving diphenoxylate (Lomotil) should be altered to the following side effect related to this medication:
    a. anxiety
    b. bradycardia
    *c. drowsiness
    d. urinary retention

5. The following medication is used to treat the diarrhea associated with bacillary dysentery caused by *Shigella* organisms:
    *a. ampicillin (Omnipen)
    b. cholestyramine (Questran)
    c. kaolin (Donnagel)
    d. psyllium preparations (Metamucil)

CHAPTER 63

1. An over-the-counter medication used to treat nausea is
   *a. Emetrol
   b. Reglan
   c. Phenergan
   d. Ativan

2. The following symptom may be related to the use of dronabinol (Marinol):
   a. bradycardia
   b. hypertension
   c. rash
   *d. anxiety

3. Persons taking phenothiazines need to be assessed for extrapyramidal symptoms, which include
   a. dysphoria, drowsiness, and dizziness
   *b. dyskinesia, dystonia, and akathisia
   c. dry mouth, blurred vision, and urinary retention
   d. hypotension, confusion, and shuffling gait

4. Your client is to receive metoclopramide (Reglan) for nausea. The following statement by your client leads you to believe that she has understood the teaching that you have done:
   a. "During episodes of nausea, I will drink clear liquids."
   *b. "I may be drowsy as a result of taking this medication."
   c. "This medication should be taken on a full stomach."
   d. "I will need to take supplemental potassium while I am taking this medication."

5. Before administering an antiemetic to a patient experiencing nausea and vomiting, the nurse should assess
   a. blood pressure
   b. heart rate
   c. weight
   *d. bowel sounds

6. Prochlorperazine (Compazine) is contraindicated in
   a. children under the age of 12 years
   b. preoperative patients
   *c. pregnant women
   d. persons under 100 pounds

7. Which of the following antiemetics is the drug of choice for use with children?
   *a. promethazine (Phenergan)
   b. benzquinamide (Emete-Con)
   c. buclizine (Bucladin-S)
   d. cyclizine (Marezine)

8. Mr. P is going on an ocean cruise and asks his physician for an antiemetic. Which of the following medications would be most effective for motion sickness?
   *a. meclizine (Antivert)
   b. diphenhydramine (Benadryl)
   c. hydroxyzine (Atarax)

9. A scopolamine (Transderm Scop) patch is ordered for a terminal care patient experiencing nausea and vomiting. The following statement made by your patient leads you to believe that he or she understands how to use the patch: "I will
   a. put it on in the morning and take it off at night."
   *b. place the patch behind my ear and replace it every 3 days."
   c. place the patch on the front or back of my cheek."
   d. apply a thin layer of lotion before I apply the patch to prevent irritation."

10. When administering hydroxyzine (Vistaril), you need to assess the client for anticholinergic effects, which include
    *a. dry mouth and urinary retention
    b. hypotension and bradycardia
    c. dizziness and depression
    d. drowsiness and anorexia

CHAPTER 64

1. Cancer cells' growth rate is called
   a. anaplasia
   b. pleomorphism
   c. neoplasm
   *d. proliferation

2. An alkylating anticancer drug is
   a. fluorouracil (5-FU)
   b. doxorubicin (Adriamycin)
   *c. chlorambucil (Leukeran)
   d. vincristine (Oncovin)

3. A vesicant can
   a. cause irritation to the skin
   *b. cause extensive tissue damage
   c. only be given through a chest catheter or port
   d. be given by deep IM injection if diluted with normal saline

4. Combinations of antineoplastic medications are used to
   *a. decrease the development of cell resistance
   b. increase the length of treatment
   c. increase the quantity of each medication used
   d. decrease the side effects of each medication

5. Prior to taking an antineoplastic medication, your client begins to vomit and breaks out in a sweat. He is most likely experiencing what type of reaction?
   *a. anticipatory
   b. unpredictable
   c. hypersensitive
   d. adverse

6. A cell-cycle–nonspecific medication used for the treatment of cancer is
   a. asparaginase (Elspar)
   b. hydroxyurea (Hydrea)
   c. busulfan (Myleran)
   *d. dacarbazine (DTIC-Dome)

7. The nursing diagnosis that is a priority for Mrs. P., who has stomatitis secondary to the administration of chemotherapeutic agents, is
   a. impaired skin integrity
   *b. high risk for infection
   c. alteration in nutrition
   d. high risk for bleeding

8. The following drug, if administered with mercaptopurine (Purinethol), will increase its effect:
   *a. allopurinol (Zyloprim)
   b. furosemide (Lasix)

   c. propranolol (Inderal)
   d. verapamil (Calan)

9. When administering bleomycin (Blenoxane), the nurse should assess the client for
   a. tachycardia and hypertension
   b. confusion
   c. seizures
   *d. stomatitis and alopecia

CHAPTER 65

1. A common eye disorder that may be caused by allergens, bacteria or viral infections, or chemical irritants is
   a. hordeolum
   b. blepharitis
   *c. conjunctivitis
   d. glaucoma

2. Corneal ulcers are most frequently caused by
   a. injury by vegetative matter
   *b. bacterial infections
   c. fungal infections following steroid therapy
   d. inadequate lacrimation

3. Autonomic ophthalmic drops are used
   *a. for diagnostic and therapeutic purposes
   b. to treat fungal infections
   c. to treat inflammatory infections
   d. to reduce intraocular pressure

4. Long-term use of ophthalmic corticosteroids may result in
   a. pseudodiabetes
   *b. glaucoma
   c. weight gain
   d. hypokalemia

5. A small device inserted into the conjunctival area that releases pilocarpine is
   a. fluorescein
   b. retrobulbar injection
   *c. Ocusert
   d. sub Tenon's injection

6. When administering eye drops, you should pull the
   *a. lower lid down and drop the medication in the conjunctival sac
   b. lower lid down and drop the medication on the eye, being careful not to touch it with the applicator
   c. upper lid up and have the person look down
   d. upper lid up and place the medication in the middle of the eye

7. Your client with glaucoma is started on dipivefrin (Propine) 1 gtt q12h. Your instructions should include the following information:
   *a. "When you take this, you may experience redness, burning, and tearing."
   b. "Nausea and anorexia are common side effects of this medication."
   c. "Lie down for 5 min and keep your eyes closed after taking the medication."
   d. "If you experience headaches, decrease the dose to once a day."

8. Cholinergic miotics reduce intraocular pressure by
   a. contracting the sphincter muscle of the eye
   b. preventing ciliary muscle spasm
   c. decreasing production of aqueous humor
   *d. increasing outflow of aqueous humor

9. A person receiving Diamox may experience
   *a. increased volume and frequency of urination
   b. increased sputum and bronchoconstriction
   c. nausea and paresthesia
   d. hypertension and dysrhythmias

10. Pilocarpine (Pilocar) causes
    *a. miosis
    b. mydriasis
    c. no pupillary change
    d. diplopia

11. The following statement demonstrates that the client understands the teaching that you have done regarding pilocarpine:
    a. "I know that I must eat foods high in potassium and stay away from salt."
    *b. "I know that I will have decreased vision in dim light, so I do not plan to drive at night."
    c. "The dosage of pilocarpine will need to be increased as I get older."

d. "I can no longer operate heavy machinery."

12. Lubricants are used for
    a. conjunctivitis
    b. blepharitis
    *c. keratitis
    d. corneal ulcers

13. A dye used to diagnose lesions or foreign bodies in the eye is
    a. atropine
    b. mannitol
    c. dexamethasone
    *d. fluorescein

14. A client receiving timolol (Timoptic) should be instructed about the adverse effects of the medication which include
    *a. ocular burning
    b. drooping eyelids
    c. swelling around the eye
    d. decreased peripheral vision

15. The following medication is used in newborns to prevent eye damage from gonorrhea:
    a. cromolyn sodium
    b. Mannitol
    c. silver nitrate
    *d. erythromycin

16. The following medication should be questioned if it is ordered for a client with glaucoma:
    a. Demerol
    b. Vistaril
    *c. atropine
    d. gentamicin

17. Acute angle-closure glaucoma may be evidenced as
    a. watery, mucoid discharge
    b. pressure and dull pain which radiates to the face
    *c. sudden severe pain
    d. redness, edema, heat, and tenderness

CHAPTER 66

1. Mrs. J. states that she applies Neosporin ointment to every cut that her son gets. Identify the best reply to Mrs. J's statement:

   a. "Lesions can occur with chronic use of Neosporin."

   b. "That is an excellent idea; it will prevent your son from developing an infection."

   *c. "Drug resistance can develop with overuse of topical antibiotics."

   d. "When the skin is broken, more of the drug is absorbed systemically, so you need to observe for toxic side effects of the medication."

2. One of the most effective topical agents for acne is

   a. Neosporin

   *b. benzoyl peroxide

   c. chlorhexidine (Hibiclens)

   d. pHisoHex

3. Mrs. P. is applying cornstarch to J. J.'s perineal area every time she changes his diaper. What instructions will you give her?

   *a. cornstarch may promote growth of bacteria and fungi

   b. cornstarch is very drying to the skin, only use it when J.J. has a rash

   c. cornstarch should be applied no more than 4 times a day

   d. apply the cornstarch on J.J.'s diaper, not directly to his skin

4. The physician orders tretinoin (Retin-A) for a client's acne. The following instructions should be given to her:

   a. "You should see positive results from the medication within 1 week."

   b. "Wash your face before each application and use it in the morning and at bedtime."

   c. "You should leave the medication on for an hour, then remove it with soap and water."

   *d. "Apply the medication no more than once a day; overuse will cause severe inflammation."

5. Your client is using isotretinoin (Accutane) for severe acne. The following statement leads you to believe that she has understood your teaching:

   a. "I will increase my intake of foods high in vitamin K."

   *b. "I will avoid extended exposure to direct sunlight."

   c. "I will wash my face four time a day and apply the medication after each washing."

   d. "After 4–6 weeks of using this drug, my acne should clear up."

6. B. H. has a rash in his axillae. His physician prescribes a topical corticosteroid. An adverse effect of excessive administration of topical steroids is

   *a. atrophy of the skin

   b. superinfection

   c. cracking and splitting of the skin

   d. loss of pigmentation in the area of application

7. The following agent is the drug of choice for treating psoriasis:

   *a. acitretin

   b. acetic acid

   c. gentian violet

   d. sulfur

8. P. G. has been exposed to poison ivy. Which of the following medications would be most helpful to relieve her itching?

   a. coal tar (Balnetar)

   *b. colloidal oatmeal (Aveeno)

   c. trioxsalen (Trisoralen)

   d. sutilains (Travase)

9. Mr. J. is being treated with isotretinoin (Accutane) for severe acne. The nurse should assess Mr. J. for which of the following adverse responses to the medication?

   *a. nausea, vomiting, and blurred vision

   b. hypertension and arrhythmias

   c. hair loss

   d. anorexia and diarrhea

10. The following statement by Mr. R. leads you to believe that he has understood the teaching that you have done regarding Halotex for athlete's feet. "I will

    a. apply the ointment daily for 6 weeks."

    b. use the powder 3 times a day and only wear white socks for the next month."

    c. soak my feet in cold water before each application."

    *d. apply the medication at morning and bed time for 2–4 weeks."

11. Astringents are used
    a. to relieve pruritus and dry skin
    *b. for their drying effects on exudative lesions
    c. to debride wounds
    d. for removal of necrotic tissue

12. Antibiotics available in topical form for acne include
    a. neomycin and vancomycin
    b. penicillin and Rocephin
    *c. clindamycin and erythromycin
    d. bacitracin and polymyxin B

CHAPTER 67

1. You should observe a client receiving a magnesium infusion for the following:
    a. dry pale skin
    *b. hyporeflexia
    c. agitation
    d. increase respirations

2. In the event that a client receiving magnesium sulfate demonstrates symptoms related to hypermagnesemia, you should be prepared to administer
    a. oxygen
    b. epinephrine
    c. potassium phospate
    *d. calcium gluconate

3. The following outcome would indicate successful management of preeclampsia with magnesium sulfate
    a. decreased contractions
    b. respiratory rate less than 16 hours
    *c. absence of seizure activity
    d. absent reflexes

4. You should be aware that administration of meperidine during labor can result in
    a. reduction in signs of fetal stress
    b. fetal hyperactivity
    *c. prolongation of the latent stage of labor
    d. uterine tetany

5. During ritodrine administration for premature labor, the nurse will
    *a. auscultate heart sounds frequently
    b. maintain the client on her left side
    c. encourage activity and range-of-motion exercises
    d. provide small frequent meals

Testbank Data Disk Instructions

For use on IBM PC compatibles and Macintosh systems (with or without WINDOWS) equipped with a Super Drive

INTRODUCTION

This electronic test-generating program contains plain .RTF word-processing files for the

Instructor's Manual and Testbank by Anne Collins Abrams and Gail Ropelewski-Ryan, to accompany Clinical Drug Therapy: *Rationales for Nursing Practice*, sixth edition, by Anne Collins Abrams

Test items for each chapter are stored in separate files and all ANSWERS appear together in ONE file. For example, test items for Chapter 7 can be found under the file name that would include the number "7" or "07". Disk files can be used with any commercial word processing software. The files mirror the printed version (if applicable) with the exception that underlined (or italicized) material is roman and subscripts and superscripts may not ascend or descend. For example, CO_2 may appear as CO2. You will have to use your own word processor to make necessary adjustments. You may also use test items as is, or you may alter them in accordance with your own specifications.

HARDWARE AND SOFTWARE REQUIREMENTS

Word processing software for the IBM PC (or compatible) or Macintosh systems complete with memory and include hardware necessary to run any type of word processing software.

INSTRUCTIONS

Before using any of the files on disk, make a copy of the master disk onto a new **formatted** blank disk by opening your word processing program and copying files as you normally would. (You may have to copy files to your hard drive before making an additional disk copy.

If your word processor has a **Text IN/OUT** feature, you should use this when loading files because they are stored in generic .RTF (DOS) text file format and would be much easier to use. Otherwise, retrieve them exactly the same as you would any other document on a disk.

1. To use actual Testbank files, start your word-processing software as you normally would and re-set your margins. You **must** use your own word processing software in order to be able to view or "edit" files.

2. Files may be stored with a hard return at the end of every line. If you plan to add, delete, or change text within a line, you will need to use your backspace key to delete any hard returns in the surrounding text or search and remove them. Your word-processing software can then wrap words from one line to another *automatically* based on your margin set-up.

3. When you have modified files, save them on a separate blank **formatted** disk. For preservation, do *not* re-save any documents you've altered on the original Testbank disk(s).